# Ready for Birth & Baby

## Class Manual

*By Patty Brennan*

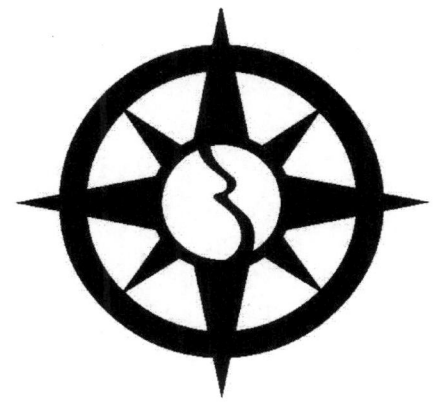

*Guidance, education and inspiration
for expectant parents …*

**Presented by**

# Center for the Childbearing Year, LLC
## www.center4cby.com

*Ready for Birth & Baby Class Manual* is available for purchase from Center for the Childbearing Year [www.center4cby.com]. A 40% wholesale discount is available for orders of six or more copies of a book.

ISBN 978-1530959594

# Table of Contents

**PREGNANCY TOPICS**

**LABOR & BIRTH TOPICS**

**POSTPARTUM TOPICS**

# Pregnancy Topics

# Early Choices Matter—Choice of Caregiver and Place of Birth
## Best of the Web

### The Birth Facts
www.thebirthfacts.com
Links to evidence-based maternity care; numerous helpful articles

### BirthNetwork National
www.birthnetwork.org
***Provider Guide.*** Encourages consumers to seek providers who support their personal philosophy of birth and allows you to create custom searches for a provider. (Only providers who have endorsed the Coalition to Improve Maternity Services' (CIMS) *Mother-Friendly Childbirth Initiative* are listed.) You can also search for a BirthNetwork chapter in your area, many of which hold monthly meetings where you can get even more valuable information about local birth options. Also publishes an online ***Birth and Beyond: A Resource Guide***

### The Birth Survey (from CIMS)
www.thebirthsurvey.com
*The Birth Survey* is an on-going, online consumer survey that asks women to provide feedback about their birth experience with a particular doctor or midwife and within a specific birth environment. Responses are made available online to other women who are deciding where and with whom to birth. Paired with this experiential data are official statistics from state departments of health listing obstetrical intervention rates at the facility level.

### Center for the Childbearing Year
www.center4cby.com
- Midwifery in Michigan: A Consumer's Guide
- What is a Doula? A Consumer's Guide to Getting the Help You Need
- Download our Free Sample Pack & Demos that includes a short online class, *Choices in Childbirth a Consumer's Guide* for more information on this important topic.

### Childbirth Connection
www.childbirthconnection.org
This website is a trustworthy source for up-to-date, evidence-based information and resources on planning for pregnancy, labor and birth, and the postpartum period. Childbirth Connection is a national nonprofit organization dedicated to improving the quality and value of maternity care through consumer engagement and health system transformation. See:

***Choosing a Caregiver: What You Need to Know***
- Why is choosing a caregiver one of the most important maternity decisions I will make?

- How will my choice of caregiver influence where I can give birth?
- What are important considerations when choosing a maternity caregiver?
- What are some insufficient reasons for choosing a caregiver?
- How do types of caregivers differ from one another?
- What if I change my mind and want to switch to another caregiver?

## Coalition to Improve Maternity Services (CIMS)

www.motherfriendly.org

CIMS is a coalition of individuals and national organizations with concern for the care and wellbeing of mothers, babies and families. Their mission is to promote a wellness model of maternity care that will improve birth outcomes and substantially reduce costs. This evidence-based mother-, baby-, and family-friendly model focuses on prevention and wellness as alternatives to high-cost screening, diagnosis and treatment programs. See ***The Mother-Friendly Childbirth Initiative*** and ***Evidence Basis for the Ten Steps of Mother-Friendly Care (PDF).***

## Lamaze International

www.lamaze.org

***Six Healthy Birth Practices***. The six practices below are supported by research studies that examine the benefits and risks of maternity care practices. They represent "evidence-based care," which is the gold standard for maternity care worldwide. Evidence-based care means using the best research about the effects of specific procedures, drugs, tests and treatments to help guide decision-making. PDF files summarizing the evidence in support of the six practices can be found on the Lamaze International website.

1. *Let Labor Begin on Its Own*
2. *Walk, Move Around, and Change Positions Throughout Labor*
3. *Bring a Loved One, Friend, or Doula for Continuous Support*
4. *Avoid Interventions that are Not Medically Necessary*
5. *Avoid Giving Birth on Your Back and Follow Your Body's Urges to Push*
6. *Keep Mother and Baby Together—It's Best for Mother, Baby, and Breastfeeding*

## Waterbirth International

www.waterbirth.org

Frequently asked questions, benefits of, research, pool information and more.

# Folic Acid

Folic acid is a B vitamin that can help prevent birth defects of the brain and spinal cord called neural tube defects (NTDs). Folic acid works to prevent these birth defects only if taken before conception and during early pregnancy.

Because NTDs originate in the first month of pregnancy, before many women know they are pregnant, it is important for a woman to have enough folic acid in her system before conception. Folic acid is recommended for all women of childbearing age because about half of all pregnancies in this country are unplanned. Studies show that if all women consumed the recommended amount of folic acid before and during early pregnancy, up to 70 percent of all NTDs could be prevented. An estimated 3,000 pregnancies in the United States are affected by NTDs each year, most commonly spina bifida and anencephaly. Folic acid may also help prevent prematurity and other birth defects, including cleft lip and palate and some heart defects.

**How much folic acid does a woman need?**
The March of Dimes recommends that all women who can become pregnant take a multivitamin that contains at least 400 micrograms of folic acid every day starting before pregnancy, as part of a healthy diet. Folate is the natural form of folic acid that is found in certain foods including leafy green vegetables, dried beans, legumes, oranges and orange juice. Cooking and storage can destroy some of the folate in foods.

Folic acid from vitamin supplements and fortified foods is more readily absorbed and made available for use by the body than natural folate from food. The body absorbs about 50 percent of food folate. By contrast, the body absorbs approximately 85 percent of the folic acid in fortified foods and 100 percent of the folic acid in a vitamin supplement. Many studies have shown that the synthetic form of folic acid helps prevent NTDs. The Institute of Medicine (IOM), the Centers for Disease Control and Prevention (CDC) and the March of Dimes recommend that women who could become pregnant consume at least 400 micrograms a day of the synthetic form of folic acid.

**Do women need folic acid throughout pregnancy?**
Yes. A pregnant woman needs extra folic acid throughout pregnancy to help her produce the additional blood cells her body needs during pregnancy. Folic acid also supports the rapid growth of the placenta and fetus and is needed to produce new DNA (genetic material) as cells multiply. Without adequate amounts of folic acid, cell division could be impaired, possibly leading to poor growth in the fetus or placenta. The IOM recommends that women increase their intake of folic acid to 600 micrograms a day (from supplements and food sources) once their pregnancy is confirmed. Most health care providers recommend a prenatal vitamin. Most prenatal vitamins contain 800 to 1,000 micrograms of folic acid.

# Food Warnings

## Fish/Seafood

It's well known that eating seafood contaminated with mercury is a threat to human health and particularly to pregnant women and children. The Food and Drug Administration (FDA) warns pregnant women, nursing mothers, children and women who might become pregnant to avoid or limit eating certain species of fish due to excessively high levels of methyl mercury.

### Avoid
- Swordfish
- Shark
- Tilefish
- King mackerel
- Tuna steak

### Limit
- Canned tuna
- Sea Bass
- Gulf Coast Oysters
- Marlin
- Halibut
- Pike
- Walleye
- White Croaker
- Largemouth Bass
- Mahi Mahi
- Blue Mussels
- Cod
- Eastern Oysters
- Channel Catfish (wild)
- Great Lakes Salmon
- Gulf Coast Blue Crab
- Lake Whitefish
- Pollack

### Best Choices (The following fish/seafood are lowest in methyl mercury levels.)
- Catfish (farmed)
- Blue Crab (mid-Atlantic)
- Croaker
- Fish Sticks

- Flounder (summer)
- Haddock
- Trout (farmed)
- Salmon (wild Pacific)
- Shrimp

## Other Foods to Avoid
- Unpasteurized milk or juice
- Soft cheeses like feta and Brie
- Unheated deli meats and hot dogs
- Refrigerated, smoked seafood
- Undercooked poultry, meat or seafood
- Dolomite and bone meal (calcium supplements that contain lead, capable of causing neurologic damage)
- Food additives such as phenylalanine found in soda and preservatives, especially nitrites, found in lunch meats
- Aspartame, an artificial sweetener found in diet sodas and some dry goods (brand names NutraSweet, Equal, Spoonful and EqualMeasure); accounts for over 75 percent of adverse reactions to food additives reported to the FDA; read more about symptoms and diseases associated with its use at www.Mercola.com.

# Hazards

**Alcohol**
Fetal Alcohol Syndrome is a pattern of physical and mental defects in the baby; associated with low birth weight; a high blood-level of alcohol at any time during pregnancy is dangerous to the baby.

**Nicotine**
Harmful to the baby; associated with respiratory problems after birth and placental abnormalities that can contribute to excess maternal bleeding at the time of delivery or before. Smokers are at greater risk of miscarriage, premature birth and stillbirth. Children of heavy smokers have more health problems and are at a greater risk of sudden infant death syndrome (SIDS).

**Caffeine**
Found in coffee, tea, soda pop, chocolate and many over-the-counter drugs.

**Illegal Drugs**
All illegal drugs, such as cocaine, heroin, uppers, downers, hallucinogenics, etc. are dangerous to you and the baby.

**Over-the-Counter Drugs**
None proven safe; use non-drug alternatives instead. Aspirin affects the blood's clotting ability and may inhibit hormones that stimulate labor.

**Prescription Drugs**
Even relatively serious health problems during pregnancy can be controlled through the use of herbs and natural methods of treatment so as to avoid the detrimental side effects of most drugs. Some antibiotics are known to affect the developing teeth of the fetus, for example. Many drugs upset delicate hormonal balances in ways that are not fully understood. Consult a midwife or naturopath for alternative treatments for yeast and bladder infections, as well as common colds and flus.

**Radiation**
Avoid x-rays. The verdict is still out on non-ionizing radiation (microwaves and computer VDTs, for example), but there is some evidence that VDTs present a higher risk of miscarriage to women with high exposure.

**Toxoplasmosis**
Parasitic infection carried in cat feces. For adults it is seldom serious, but for a woman who acquires the parasite for the first time during pregnancy, can cause miscarriage or birth defects. Stay away from cat litter boxes, raw or undercooked meats, garden soil and sand boxes.

### Heat
Body temperature over 102 degrees in first trimester is associated with fetal deformities. Avoid prolonged exposure to heat such as saunas and hot tubs that raise core body temperature.

### Household Chemicals
Avoid lawn care chemicals, pesticides, insecticides, herbicides, hair dyes, permanents, turpentine, paint strippers, spray adhesives and soaps with hexachlorophene. If redoing an older house, be alert to the possibility of asbestos and lead dust and leave the work to someone else.

### Electromagnetic Fields
Electric blankets and heated waterbeds are associated with more than 7x the number of miscarriages and birth defects.

# Potential Danger Signs

Call your care provider promptly if you experience any of the following symptoms while pregnant:

- ✓ Vaginal bleeding
- ✓ Persistent, severe vomiting
- ✓ Frequent burning urination
- ✓ High fever
- ✓ Steady abdominal pain or painful, persistent cramping (may be felt in the back)
- ✓ Sudden escape of fluid from the vagina (sometimes confused with loss of bladder control; the pH of fluid can be checked if you are not sure whether it is urine or amniotic fluid)
- ✓ Loss of, or significant decrease in baby's activity
- ✓ Severe diarrhea lasting longer than 48 hours

# Signs of Premature Labor

## Definition

Preterm or premature labor happens when you go into labor before 37 completed weeks of pregnancy. This is too early for your baby to be born. Babies born too soon can have lifelong or life-threatening health problems.

## Symptoms

- ✓ Contractions every 10 minutes or more often
- ✓ Change in vaginal discharge
- ✓ Pelvic pressure
- ✓ Low, dull backache
- ✓ Cramps that feel like your period
- ✓ Abdominal cramps with or without diarrhea

## Can preterm labor be stopped?

Many women are given drugs to try to delay or stop preterm labor. In some cases, birth can be delayed long enough to transport mom to a hospital with a neonatal intensive care unit. Women may also be given medications that can improve the baby's health, even if the baby comes early.

## What should you do if you think you're having preterm labor?

Call your health care provider or go to the hospital right away if you think you're having preterm labor or if you have any of the warning signs. Call even if you have only one sign. Your health care provider may tell you to:

- ✓ Come into the office or go to the hospital for a checkup.
- ✓ Stop what you're doing and rest on your left side for one hour.
- ✓ Drink 2–3 glasses of water or juice (not coffee or soda).

If the symptoms get worse or do not go away after one hour, call your provider again or go to the hospital. If the symptoms get better, relax for the rest of the day.

# Pre-Eclampsia

Pre-eclampsia is one of the major complications of pregnancy and is one reason why regular prenatal care is so important. Also known as toxemia, eclampsia is life threatening for both mom and baby. Some researchers (see especially the work of Dr. Thomas Brewer) have found a connection between pre-eclampsia and a lack of adequate protein in the diet.

At each prenatal visit, your midwife or doctor will take your blood pressure and check your urine to see whether it is positive for protein. Symptoms of sudden, severe edema (or swelling) of ankles, hands and face may also be present in the woman who is developing pre-eclampsia.

Women should be aware of the early signs of pre-eclampsia (toxemia is the later, convulsive and life-threatening stage of the disease). Talk to your midwife or doctor if you notice any of the following symptoms:

- Constipation lasting longer than 48 hours. At least one good bowel movement per day is desirable to assure that the body is eliminating toxins efficiently.
- Sudden, excessive weight gain (10 pounds in 3 days)
- Severe, continuous headaches
- Dimness or blurred vision
- Swelling of face and/or fingers
- Persistent vomiting
- Decrease in urine output

Late Symptoms:

- Epigastric pain (sharp pain under the ribs)
- Convulsions

# Fetal Movement Counting

One way to check your baby's health before birth is to count the number of times he or she moves in a certain period each day. This number is the fetal movement count. Babies do not move constantly. They may sleep and then wake up and move. Your midwife or doctor may recommend that you count fetal movements at some point in late pregnancy, due to the presence of a specific risk factor, or you may notice a change in movement on your own that you find concerning. Here is a way to check in with your baby.

## How to Record Fetal Movements

- Choose the time of day when your baby is most active.
- Rest on your left or right side. Get in a comfortable position.
- You may want to eat or drink something before counting fetal movements; food can make your baby more active.
- Your baby may be more active if you move around shortly before doing counts.
- Do not smoke; smoking is harmful to you and your baby and may make your baby less active for up to 90 minutes.
- Count all of your baby's movements—kicks, rolls, and big and little movements; sometimes you can see a ripple or little bump on your abdomen when the baby changes position; some women describe the movements as rolling, stretching or pushing; each feeling of movement counts as one movement.
- If you cannot feel your baby moving on the inside, place your hands lightly on your belly and watch for movement.
- Look at a clock and write down the time you start counting.
- Each time the baby moves make a mark on the paper.
- **When you have counted 10 movements in an hour, stop counting; this is reassuring.**
- If the baby moved less than 8–10 times in an hour, count the movements for another hour.

If you would like to use a chart to keep track of your fetal movement count, simply Google "fetal movement count" and the results will yield a variety of tools.

Call your midwife or doctor if there are still less than 8–10 movements in the second hour of timing.

Call your midwife or doctor if you notice a big change in movement. Tell him/her when you last felt your baby move and if the movement changed slowly or suddenly. Your midwife or doctor may use other ways to check the baby such as listening to the baby's heart rate or monitoring the heart rate pattern over time.

# Prenatal Nutrition Overview

I've never been one for counting calories and grams or micrograms of this nutrient and that one. Quantitative nutritional information abounds in the literature and tends to be the focus of what passes for nutritional advice for pregnant and breastfeeding mothers. It doesn't strike me as particularly useful or applicable. I mean, unless we are on a diet, do any of us really measure everything we put in our mouths? And wouldn't it be rather obsessive-compulsive if we did?

Rather, let's emphasize a common sense approach that sidesteps the ever-present food pyramid, charts and tables. The cornerstone of this approach is "how do you feel?" A few tables and numbers are given, not for rigid adherence purposes, but to use as a baseline, to see if you are in the ballpark, so to speak. Our focus will be on qualitative information, basic principles and a few simple ideas. What does your body need to grow a healthy baby and ensure that, in the process, you maintain good energy levels and do not become depleted or suffer symptoms related to deficiencies and poor nutritional choices? First, let's address some of the abundant myths.

**Myth:** Salt intake causes you to retain fluid in your system, leading to swelling of ankles and feet, and should therefore be minimized, if not eliminated, during pregnancy.

**Fact:** Salt is an essential inorganic constituent of body cells and tissues and regulates fluid balance in the system. It is a component of blood. During pregnancy, the mother's blood volume expands by almost 50 percent! Salt is needed to help build the blood supply, so go ahead and salt your food to taste. To increase the nutritional value of your salt, use sea salt (as all of the minerals have been removed from common table salt and kosher salt). If your ankles are swelling, make sure you are drinking enough fluids (see more on this subject below) and cut out foods high in chemical preservatives, especially nitrites (such as found in lunch meats and other highly-processed meats).

**Myth:** Fats make you fat.

**Fact:** Excess carbohydrate intake spikes the blood sugar and sends a message to the pancreas to produce more insulin (the fat-storing hormone). Fats actually slow down the absorption of carbohydrates in the bloodstream as well as helping the system to digest protein. If you're worried about excess weight gain, focus instead on stabilizing your blood sugar by limiting intake of refined carbs (white flour products, sugar and junk food); eating healthy carbs (a variety of whole grains, fresh fruits and vegetables); controlling the quantity of food eaten at a meal; and eating a moderate amount of satisfying, high-quality fats with your meals.

A lot has been written on the difference between "good" fats and the "bad," trans, or polyunsaturated fats. See more below.

**Myth:** Animal fats are bad for you.

**Fact:** The opposite is true. Animal fats are good for you! (Check out the publications of the Weston A. Price Foundation, in particular, Sally Fallon's book, *Nourishing Traditions.*) The single most important dietary influence for prenatal nutrition is adequate omega-3 fats. Flax seeds, walnuts and other plant sources of omega-3 should not be substituted for animal omega3s as you will simply not receive the same benefits due to intrinsic metabolic inefficiencies. The human organism will struggle to create a perfectly formed brain and needed hormones without animal fat. Allow yourself to eat butter, cream and eggs, along with fish (in moderation), meat and, if you like it, liver. Contrary to popular belief, the truth is that these fats (especially from healthy, clean sources) are essential, satisfying and delicious.

It is true, however, that the meat industry in the U.S. is rife with unhealthy practices involving contaminated, chemicalized feed for the animals; crowded, unsanitary and inhumane living conditions; and extensive use of hormones, antibiotics and other drugs added to the animals' feed to stimulate unnatural growth and combat the horrible living conditions—all in pursuit of making money at all costs. Free-range, organic, grass-fed animals on the other hand, produce a very healthy source of food. Many small farmers are rising to the occasion, providing healthy, bio-dynamic meat and dairy products for those who want them. Admittedly, clean sources of meat and dairy are more expensive, so what may be "ideal" must be balanced with the realities of your pocketbook.

If you follow a vegan diet and are unwilling to eat animal fats of any kind, do your best to consume good quality fats from non-animal sources such as coconut, olive and flaxseed oils; avocados; nuts and seeds; and be sure to take a vitamin B12 supplement.

**Myth:** Pregnant women need 100 grams of protein per day.

**Fact:** That's a lot of protein! Any woman I have ever worked with who was trying to stick to the "Brewer Diet," struggled to comply with the recommendation, typically complaining about feeling too full and not really having an appetite that matched the regimen. Pregnant women do require extra protein throughout the day, it is true. But rigid adherence to a 100-grams-of-protein daily regimen is quite likely to end in digestive stress, excessive weight gain and a big baby. Rather than focusing on quantity, emphasize quality sources of protein from clean, organic sources if possible. Avoid over-dependence on packaged lunch meats, for example, which are loaded with chemical preservatives, and substitute sliced fresh chicken or turkey breast instead. Your kidneys and liver will thank you. These organ systems, after all, are working double hard to purify your bloodstream and eliminate waste from your body. They don't need extra toxins thrown into the mix.

If you are pregnant with twins or multiples, or were under-nourished when you became pregnant, then extra protein, up to 100 grams per day even, may be beneficial. Sudden growth spurts of the baby may stimulate an appetite for more protein, specific nutrients, or more calories overall.

Trust your body's signals and give it what it needs. 100 grams of protein a day is not wrong; it is just not necessary throughout the entire pregnancy.

**Myth:** Vitamin pills are a good source of essential vitamins and minerals.

**Fact:** Your body is designed to optimize assimilation of vitamins and minerals from food sources. Vitamin pills and supplements may have their place, but the closer they are to food sources, the more easily digested. Read labels on your prenatal vitamins. If you don't recognize the list of ingredients as foods, go to your local health food store and ask for a "food grown prenatal vitamin." They cost more, but since they digest more easily, you may be able to spread out your supply over a longer period of time and, in the end, come out about the same budget wise. If your diet is based on a variety of whole foods and you are drinking the Pregnancy Tea (see p. 27) on a fairly regular basis, then you may be able to limit pill intake to times of stress when you aren't cooking regularly (such as during illness, moving to a new home, going on vacation or overworking). Two brands that I recommend are Megafoods and New Chapter prenatal vitamins.

If your vitamins are making you feel terrible—constipation, digestive discomfort—your body is telling you that it cannot digest the pills. This means they are not really providing the purported benefits and a better means of covering your bases should be sought. If insurance is paying for your vitamin pills, then ask your care provider to write you a script for a more easily digestible vitamin.

## Guiding Principles for Healthy Eating During Pregnancy

### Drink More Fluids

This is a key concept, important not only during pregnancy, but in labor and birth, and during the early weeks and months postpartum as well. Remember that meeting minimal recommendations is not the same as optimal and may be insufficient if you are losing a lot of fluid through sweating or due to an illness that includes symptoms such as fever, diarrhea or vomiting.

> Recommended Daily Fluid Intake during Pregnancy
>
> your body weight ÷ 2 = # fluid ounces per day

During pregnancy, extra fluid is needed to properly expand the blood volume which, in turn, infuses the placenta with nutrients for your baby. You are also creating amniotic fluid, which constantly replenishes itself. In labor, extra fluid is needed because you are working hard, sweating, possibly leaking amniotic fluid or vomiting, and may be doing lots of mouth breathing, all of which can lead to dehydration. After labor, you need to replace lost fluids, including normal blood loss, make breast milk, and help your system flush out the now superfluous systemic fluids that supported your growing baby. "Drink more fluids" is a consistent through throughout the childbearing year. Consciousness about it and developing new habits and ways of eating will help you feel your best.

**What are the signs that you are not getting enough fluid?**

- Urine may be deeply colored, appear concentrated, have a strong odor and be reduced in frequency and amount. Look for urine to be pale yellow as a sign that you are drinking sufficient quantities. Be aware that some vitamin supplements (such as B vitamins) may color the urine to a bright yellow so that color may not be a reliable indicator in all cases.

- Mucous membranes and skin may be dry.

- Constipation, especially when accompanied by a toxic headache.

- Swelling in the extremities may indicate that your body is holding on to extra fluids because it has gotten the wrong message. The only problem here is that the cell walls are breaking down and fluid is leaving the bloodstream where it is needed, seeping out into interstitial tissues. Drink more fluids and non-pathological swelling should go down while urine output increases.

- Muscle contractions, including uterine contractions. **Dehydration can cause premature labor!** Experiencing excessive amounts contractions weeks before your due date? Consider your activities, fluid intake and environmental factors such as excessive heat in the hours leading up to the onset of contractions or uterine irritability. A call to your midwife or doctor will likely result in the recommendation to get off your feet, drink a pint of fluid and call back in an hour if contractions continue unabated. If dehydration is the cause, the midwife's simple prescription will likely resolve the problem. However, do not hesitate to seek medical care if contractions continue.

- Under-production or decrease in the milk supply.

- **Warning:** Severe vomiting and diarrhea or high fever during pregnancy may require medical treatment. Call your doctor or midwife and follow his/her advice. I have seen cases of food poisoning and flu lead to premature onset of labor when administration of intravenous fluids could have prevented the problem.

### Vitamins and Minerals
Pregnant women need increased quantities of all vitamins and minerals. There are two minerals which are especially important—iron and calcium, and each is discussed in depth below.

### Weight Gain
Try not to worry so much about this! A healthy weight gain is likely to be between 25 and 40 pounds for most women. If you have little to no fat on your body going into the pregnancy, then it may be desirable for you to gain more than the minimum 25 pounds. Your body will naturally want to lay down a fat reserve for breastfeeding which requires more daily calories than needed

to grow the baby in utero. If you are overweight when you first become pregnant (by objective medical standards, not insane fashion model standards), then you can shoot for a minimum weight gain of 20 pounds. BUT, give up empty junk food calories and sweets and never go hungry. If you have a tendency to obsess about the scale, consider giving up your scale addiction and going with this idea—if your arms and thighs are getting thinner as your belly grows, then you are not taking in enough calories. Celebrate your growing curves and softness, your essential feminine self!

To avoid the "I gained 10 pounds with each pregnancy that I never lost syndrome" you need to recognize that it's time to reign it in a bit and go back to your pre-pregnant calorie intake when your baby starts to get non-mom sources of nutrition (but not before!), typically between 6 and 8 months for breastfeeding moms. The challenge here is that you have now developed a 15-month-long habit of purposefully eating more food. Recognize that it is time to cultivate new habits (again) and that your body may give you mixed signals as it is readjusting. In addition, new motherhood throws many of us off former exercise regimens, usually due to lack of personal time. Look for ways to integrate the baby into a new regimen that works for you both.

**A Word about Cravings**

Cravings are simply information from your body. Step outside yourself a moment and read the message. Your body is telling you what you need. Cravings for eggs (little protein bombs) or milk are not unusual. Try following your cravings. If you are a vegetarian and you are having dreams about a rare steak, you don't necessarily need to give in to the craving which you might find gross. But you do need to find a way to meet your increased need for protein. If you crave dairy products but can't digest them well, then look for non-dairy sources of calcium and protein. Meet the true need and the craving should diminish.

If your cravings are for caffeine or sugar and you are accustomed to feeding this craving, then you may be under the influence of an addiction. Try this instead—observe the pattern of your craving. Do you crave something sweet or a comfort food at the same time each day, say 11am or 3pm or 9pm (between meals)? Are there physical symptoms that precede or accompany this craving such as nausea, light-

> Addictions are the one exception to the "follow your cravings" rule.

headedness, or sinking energy? Or are you simply in the habit of having something sweet at this time of day? Which is it? Feeding the sugar craving will further de-stabilize your blood sugar and increase your symptoms, enabling you to feel better quickly as your blood sugar rises, but leading to another crash when the spike is over. A proactive high-protein snack before the expected crash should prevent the low blood sugar that is causing your symptoms while helping to stabilize your energy levels throughout the day. On the other hand, if you simply require a treat before bedtime, go for it (but give a whole grain, naturally sweetened treat a chance).

Your relationship with food has changed for the foreseeable future. Make peace with it! Old strategies of skipping breakfast, grabbing something quick (and sweet) on the go, fueling yourself with coffee, and so on, will no longer serve you well (if they ever truly did!). During pregnancy, the body becomes more sensitive. Another person is involved in your choices. *Hunger is an urgent experience, not something to be ignored and pushed past.* Think of it as preparation for parenthood. New bio-rhythms are taking hold and food has just become a whole lot more important (as the mother of any newborn, toddler or child knows). It will take some planning and, going forward, there is no such option as an empty refrigerator or skipping breakfast. That said, a little planning will go a long way. You don't have to become a fabulous whole foods cook. Packaged foods (yogurt, hummus, trail mix) or pieces of fresh fruit will work just fine if you have them on hand.

A bowl of oatmeal (make it instant if you must) or a couple of eggs with whole grain toast and a piece of fresh fruit for breakfast can be followed up by a handful (or two) of trail mix, an apple, and a glass of milk mid-morning. A hearty bowl of soup, a sandwich, or salad with protein serves as a satisfying lunch. To keep blood sugar levels even through to dinner time, try some hummus dip with fresh veggies and chips or cheese and crackers for an afternoon snack. And then enjoy some meat, fish or legumes with fresh veggies and brown rice or potatoes for dinner. Add a glass of milk and a whole-grain muffin or a bowl of yogurt and fruit before bed if you like. And all the while, make it all taste delicious with high-quality fats and salt to taste, and keep your water and Pregnancy Tea (see p. 27) readily available.

---

Tips for the Busy Working Pregnant Woman

✓ Quality over quantity
✓ Never go hungry
✓ Eat more frequently
✓ Plan ahead
✓ Have high-protein snacks available

---

# Protein Counting Guide

When pregnant, you will need more protein than you are likely accustomed to consuming. You may especially benefit from a high-protein breakfast each day, as well as high-protein snacks a couple of times per day. Protein, combined with complex carbohydrates, will help to stabilize your blood sugar and keep your energy levels more even throughout the day. If you have experienced a tendency to feel light-headed, even to the point of fainting, or are craving sweets, this nutritional strategy should help you feel better and avoid the hypoglycemia (low blood sugar) that is causing your symptoms.

**Dairy Products**
Milk, 1 cup, 8gm
Cheddar/Swiss Cheese 1 oz., 7gm
Cottage Cheese ½ cup, 12gm
Ice Cream 1 cup, 6gm
Yogurt 1 cup, 7gm

**Meats/ Fish/Poultry/Beans/Nuts/Seeds**
Bologna 1 oz., 3.8gm
Beef 3 oz., 20gm
Chicken 3 oz., 25gm
Egg 1, 6gm
Hot Dog 1, 7gm
Turkey 3 oz., 27gm
Pork 3 oz., 21gm
Liver 3½ oz., 26gm
Haddock 3 oz., 16gm
Salmon 3 oz., 17gm
Halibut 3½ oz., 26gm
Peanut Butter 1 tbsp., 4gm
Peanuts 1/4 cup, 9gm
Walnuts 1/4 cup, 6gm
Pinto Beans ½ cup, 7gm
Navy Beans ½ cup, 7gm
Kidney Beans ½ cup, 7gm

**Starches/Breads/Cereals**
Brown Rice 1 cup, 6gm
Corn 1 cup, 5gm
Noodles 1 cup, 6gm
Cheerios 1 1/4 cup, 3.8gm
Granola 1/4 cup, 4gm
Shredded Wheat 2/3 cup, 3gm

# Iron in Pregnancy

**Why is iron important?**

The mother's blood volume expands by nearly fifty percent to support the baby's growth. This expansion is typically completed by the beginning of the last trimester of pregnancy (approximately 28 weeks). As the volume increases, a sufficient quantity of dietary iron is required to manufacture red blood cells, the oxygen-carrying component in blood. Without it, the volume will still increase, but the blood will be relatively dilute with insufficient capacity to circulate oxygen in the system—a medical condition known as iron deficiency anemia.

**The symptoms of iron deficiency anemia are:**
- Fatigue, especially upon exertion
- Muscular weakness
- Air hunger such as huffing and puffing after climbing a flight of stairs (the body's attempt to take in more oxygen to meet the demand)
- Pallor of the mucous membranes and skin
- Orthostatic hypotension (a decrease in blood pressure when moving from a reclining to standing position, sometimes causing dizziness and/or spots before the eyes upon arising)
- Pica (cravings for non-food substances such as ice, laundry starch or clay)
- Weakened immune system
- Thin, brittle or flattened fingernails with pronounced longitudinal ridging
- Loss of sex drive

**During labor and birth, the anemic woman may experience:**
- Less effective contractions (less oxygen to uterus)
- Longer labor
- Increased experience of pain due to lactic acid build up (caused by lack of sufficient oxygen to the muscle)
- Increased risk of fetal distress as oxygen supply to baby may be compromised
- Hemorrhage due to tired uterus failing to contract normally
- Greater susceptibility to shock from normal blood loss

**After birth, the anemic mother is at greater risk of:**
- Increased risk of postpartum infection
- Low overall energy levels

**What are the causes of iron deficiency anemia?**

The primary cause during pregnancy is insufficient dietary iron to support the optimal expansion of the maternal blood volume. If a woman is borderline anemic when she became pregnant, then she will surely suffer symptoms in the absence of a concerted effort to correct the problem. Other causes are some rare diseases such as hereditary blood disorders, diseases of the bone marrow, chronic infections and internal bleeding. Contributing non-dietary causes include:

chronic diarrhea, intestinal parasites, blood donation, menstruation and the use of certain drugs such as tetracycline, neomycin or cholestramine.

**Will vitamin pills solve the problem?**

Without a conscious effort to seek out and consume iron-rich foods, most pregnant women will not consume sufficient dietary iron to meet their needs of 30–48 milligrams per day. Vitamin pills containing iron are notorious for their poor absorption rate, tendency to cause constipation and turn the stool black, and tendency to cause indigestion and gastric distress. These symptoms indicate that supplemented iron, in the form of pills, is not recognized as a food by the body and is relatively difficult to digest. So, that means that the pills are not solving the problem as intended, but rather are generating other symptoms of concern. Feel free to ditch vitamins pills that your body is rejecting as un-digestible. In other words, if your hemoglobin count is not coming up in response to supplementation, then, quite simply, what you are doing is not working.

**Iron supplements are not all equal.**

- Ferrous sulphate is commonly prescribed, despite the fact that it has poor absorbability and is associated with miscarriages, nausea, constipation and the destruction of vitamin E (which is active in preventing red blood cell death and subsequent anemia).
- Sustained-release iron pills are associated with fewer side effects but cause most of the iron to be released after it can be absorbed.
- Ferrous fumarate or ferrous gluconate may also be prescribed by your doctor or midwife and are more easily absorbed with fewer side effects.
- Chelated iron is more easily absorbed than non-chelated iron because it is chemically bonded to another substance, more easily absorbed than iron, which acts as a carrier of iron through the intestinal wall.
- Floradix Herbs Plus Iron liquid formula is a natural, food-grown source that has excellent absorbability (available at health food stores).

**A note on constipation**

Constipation is a much more serious concern during pregnancy than most medical professionals acknowledge. Few even ask the expectant mother about the regularity and ease of her bowel movements, but I believe that they should. The kidneys and liver are doing double duty during pregnancy, filtering twice the amount of blood, for both mom and baby. Ideally, the maternal system would eliminate all waste materials efficiently so as not to create a further burden for her organs. But when the system is constipated, waste materials sit in the colon and begin to reabsorb. Her organs then need to re-filter the same toxins as the blood thickens. Eventually the heart has to work harder as well. Toxic headaches may begin to manifest and the mom is now tempted to self-medicate in an effort to not feel terrible. Constipation (defined as less than one easy and satisfying bowel movement per day) should be corrected promptly and, going forward, prevented.

**Cautions:**

- Excesses of certain nutrients can cause deficiencies in others. Before taking mega doses of any supplement, seek the opinion of a healthcare provider who is knowledgeable about nutrition.
- If something is good for you, more is not necessarily better. Once a deficiency is corrected, aim for maintenance and keep an eye on your symptoms and how you are feeling.
- If you have toddlers and small children in the home, treat storage of iron supplements as you would any other medication. Excessive doses are toxic.

**Dietary Sources of Iron**

- Red meat, especially organ meats
- Clams, oysters
- Whole grains
- Bran, farina
- Beans, tofu
- Dark green leafy greens
- Nuts and seeds
- Dark molasses
- Seaweed (powdered dulse and/or kelp can be sprinkled as a salt substitute or taken in capsule form)
- Nutritional yeast
- Dried fruit
- Prune juice
- Pregnancy Tea (Nettles and Red Raspberry Leaves, prepared as an herbal infusion (see p. 27).

**To increase absorbability of dietary iron:**

- Eat high-iron foods (or iron supplements) with vitamin C or foods high in vitamin C, such as orange juice (200–500 mg of vitamin C nearly doubles iron absorption).

- Fat-soluble vitamins increase the absorbability of iron. Foods high in iron that come ready made with fat-soluble vitamins include eggs, fish, caviar, liver (especially calf's liver) and red meats. Green leafy vegetables also supply iron, although iron from animal protein is much easier to absorb. Serve leafy greens with butter and the iron is more available.

- The amount of iron absorbed decreases with increasing doses. Take prescribed daily iron supplements in two or three equally-spaced doses, preferably with food.

- Use of cast-iron cookware adds iron to food, especially if the food is acidic (tomato sauce, for example).

- Minimize exposure to cigarette smoke and other air pollutants; they rob the body of vitamin C.

- Tannic acid, caffeine and phosphates in caffeinated teas, coffee and sodas inhibit iron absorption. Space consumption of these beverages away from high-iron meals, or give them up entirely.

- Avoid antacids. Iron is better absorbed in an acid stomach; antacids neutralize stomach acids.

- Minimize use of laxatives. Laxatives decrease the length of time food remains in the upper intestine; this decreases the amount of time the body has to absorb iron.

- Minimize consumption of refined carbohydrates (sugars and white flour products). High in calories and low in nutrients, they cause the secretion of more alkaline digestive juices, thus decreasing absorbability of iron. Dairy products also neutralize stomach acids and should not be taken simultaneously with iron supplements or iron-rich foods.

- Iron-fortified foods often use a phosphate compound form of iron that is not soluble in the human digestive tract; don't count on these foods as a reliable iron source.

- Large doses of supplemental zinc or calcium can interfere with iron absorbability.

- The homeopathic cell salt Ferrum Phosphate 6X increases the assimilation of iron in the diet. Dosage is 2 tablets twice per day for up to 6 weeks.

**Remember ...**
A hemorrhage at the time of the birth is a likely cause of **postpartum anemia** for the mother. This condition will leave her susceptible to infection, low energy and depression. Focus efforts on building your blood back up with iron-rich foods, using all the strategies discussed above.

## Food Sources of Iron

| Food Source | Serving Size | Amount of Iron |
|---|---|---|
| Almonds | ¼ cup | 1.7 mg |
| Cashews | ¼ cup | 1.3 mg |
| Pistachios, shelled | ¼ cup | 2.7 mg |
| Bran flakes | ½ cup | 7.8 mg |
| Wheat bran | 3 TBSP | 4.2 mg |
| Wheat germ | 3 TBSP | 2.7 mg |
| Cream of wheat | ½ cup | 7.8 mg |
| Millet, cooked | ½ cup | 1.1 mg |
| Pumpkin or squash seeds | 2 TBSP | 3.9 mg |
| Sunflower seeds | 2 TBSP | 2.6 mg |
| Mung bean sprouts, cooked | 1 cup | 1.1 mg |
| Tofu | 4 ounces | 2.3 mg |
| Hummus | 1 TBSP | 2.9 mg |
| Miso | 3 TBSP | 1.8 mg |
| Garbanzo beans | ½ cup | 2.9 mg |
| Kidney beans | ½ cup | 3.4 mg |
| Lentils | ½ cup | 2.1 mg |
| Pinto beans | ½ cup | 3.3 mg |
| Hamburger | 3 ounces | 3.0 mg |
| Ham | 3 ounces | 2.6 mg |
| Beet greens, cooked | ½ cup | 1.9 mg |
| Spinach, cooked | ½ cup | 2.0 mg |
| Kale, cooked | ½ cup | 1.6 mg |
| Chard, cooked | ½ cup | 1.8 mg |
| Peas, cooked | ½ cup | 2.1 mg |
| Prune juice | ½ cup | 5.2 mg |
| Raisins | ¼ cup | 1.2 mg |
| Prunes | 5 medium | 1.2 mg |
| Blackstrap molasses | 1 TBSP | 3.2 mg |
| Sorghum | 1 TBSP | 2.4 mg |

# Calcium in Pregnancy

**Why is calcium important?**
Calcium is the mineral needed to create healthy bones. If mom fails to ingest sufficient amounts of dietary calcium during pregnancy, the baby's bones will be just fine as he/she will simply leach from the mother's bones the necessary nutrients. The mother, however, will be depleted and more vulnerable to a condition known as osteoporosis, a tendency for fragile bones which break easily (particularly the spinal vertebrae which may collapse, causing the hunchback noticeable in many elderly folks). So, in the end, the maternal bones are compromised by the pregnancy. If the woman has more than one pregnancy and the pattern repeats itself, the risk is increased. Then, in menopause, when bone density normally drops, vulnerability is further increased. The good news is that with a little proactive attention, this condition can be prevented!

**The symptoms of calcium deficiency are:**
A calcium deficiency during pregnancy most commonly makes itself known through muscle cramping, in particular the infamous "charley horse" or calf muscle cramp that drives the woman out of bed in the middle of the night. It can also manifest as uterine irritability.

**What is the standard medical advice given regarding calcium supplementation during pregnancy?**

- Consume dairy products, specifically 4 8-ounce glasses of whole milk per day.
- Take Tums antacids for their high-calcium.
- Take a prenatal vitamin containing 1,000 mg for women over the age of 18 and 1,300 mg for women under the age of 18.

Time constraints on many medical care providers mean that very little time is available for individualized prenatal care and proactive education. This necessitates a global, non-individualized approach to questions of diet and complaints of pregnancy. Hence the need for childbirth education to fill in this essential gap. Are there any problems with the above advice? In a word, YES. Let's consider each in turn.

**Dairy Products**
For those who can easily digest dairy products, they serve as a fine source of dietary calcium. For those who are lactose intolerant, dairy products cause gas, bloating and gastric distress and are best avoided. Calcium requirements can be met without consuming dairy products. If you find yourself craving a glass of milk, however, this is a sign from your body that you are not getting enough.

**Tums**
The form of calcium in Tums is calcium carbonate, which is not the most easily assimilated form of calcium. Cautions regarding the aluminum content of Tums have been widespread among

25

natural health advocates. GlaxoSmithKline Consumer Healthcare (the manufacturer) does not add aluminum during the manufacturing process of the TUMS tablets but one of the raw materials used in TUMS does contain negligible amounts of aluminum, measured as parts per million (ppm), ranging approximately from 100 to 500 ppm. TUMS devotees can be found on many internet pregnancy forums. Many women swear by them for relief from heartburn and indigestion. There are, however, higher-quality, more easily assimilated sources of calcium. One danger of unassimilated calcium is the tendency for kidney stones to form. Avoiding dehydration and taking all calcium supplements with food will minimize this risk.

For relief from heartburn, an alternative to TUMS is papaya enzyme tablets (dose = 4–5 tablets chewed), found at your local health food store.

### Calcium in Prenatal Vitamins

We have discussed above that humans are designed to get optimal nourishment in the form of food, not pills. While it may be comforting to read the number of milligrams of a specific nutrient contained in a pill and, therefore, be reassured that you are meeting medical recommendations, *the number on the bottle and the amount actually assimilated by your body are not necessarily equal.* Go with your symptoms. If you are suffering from nightly charley horse cramps, then you are not assimilating the calcium you are inputting. Try a better form— one that your body can digest!

## Food Sources of Calcium

| Food Source | Serving Size | Amount of Calcium |
|---|---|---|
| Whole milk | 1 cup | 292 mg |
| Low fat milk | 1 cup | 300 mg |
| Cheddar cheese | 1 ounce | 204 mg |
| Yogurt | 1 cup | 270 mg |
| Cottage cheese | 2 cup | 230 mg |
| Tofu | 4 ounces | 145 mg |
| Broccoli, cooked | 1 cup | 136 mg |
| Kale, cooked | 1 cup | 147 mg |
| Orange | 2 medium | 74 mg |
| Rhubarb, cooked | 1 cup | 211 mg |
| Almonds | ½ cup | 164 mg |
| Brazil nuts | ½ cup | 279 mg |
| Sunflower seeds | 3.5 ounces | 120 mg |
| Farina | 1 cup | 183 mg |
| Blackstrap molasses | 1 cup | 137 mg |

# Pregnancy Tea Recipe

Drinking two or three cups per day of the following herbal mixture will add substantially to the mother's health throughout pregnancy and may lessen pain and bleeding during birth. These herbs are primarily nutritive in nature (rather than medicinal), providing much-needed vitamins and minerals in a form the body can easily assimilate. Think of the herbs as dark leafy greens. The tea may be taken postpartum as well, to help tone the uterus and build a healthy milk supply. Partners can enjoy the health benefits of "Pregnancy Tea" as well. Most people find the tea mild and pleasant tasting.

**Nausea:** Do not force the tea if you are feeling averse to it due to nausea of early pregnancy. You do not want to associate it with the nausea and then be put off the idea for the rest of the pregnancy. Wait till you feel a little better and then give it a try. On the other hand, some women find that it helps, especially with a bit of Spearmint added, so it's worth a try.

**Expecting Multiples:** I have seen recommendations, by some authors, to avoid this tea when pregnant with twins. I cannot find any evidence to back up the fear that Pregnancy Tea increases the risk of premature delivery with twins. No doubt, this caution is given due to the toning effects of the Red Raspberry leaves. (It is interesting to note that calcium deficiency and dehydration, both conditions corrected by the tea, may also cause the uterus to contract.) Discuss it with your doctor or midwife and trust your instincts as to how your body may be responding to the tea. You can always drop the Red Raspberry leaves from the brew if in doubt, while still benefiting from the Nettles. Women expecting multiples have an even greater need for the extra fluids and bio-available minerals that the tea provides.

**Late Pregnancy:** If you are 36 weeks pregnant or more and have not experienced regular toning contractions (a.k.a. Braxton-Hicks contractions), then you may notice a decided effect on the uterus from drinking tea made from Red Raspberry leaves and this is recommended. Toning contractions of late pregnancy are normal.

## Ingredients

**Red Raspberry Leaves**
Contain vitamins A, B, and E, as well as calcium, phosphorous, and iron. Helps tone the uterus.

**Nettles**
The Stinging Nettle is a blood-cleansing and blood-building herb with high iron content. It is very nourishing to the kidneys and liver. Helps build a good milk supply.

**The following herbs may be added to the above mixture for variety:**

**Alfalfa**
Contains vitamins A, B12, D, E, and K, as well as calcium and phosphorous. Great for the milk supply.

**Rose Hips**
Contains the entire vitamin C complex, including bioflavonoids. Strengthening for the vascular system (hemorrhoids, varicose veins) and to boost the immune system.

**Spearmint**
Soothing to the stomach, aids in digestion, and lends a pleasant taste to the mixture. A little goes a long way.

**Red Clover**
This blood-purifying herb can be added from time to time

## Directions

Use a glass or other non-metal (aluminum is the worst) container with a lid. A wide-mouth half-gallon mason jar is perfect. Combine one part Red Raspberry leaves to one part Nettles. Add some or all of the optional herbs if desired. When using a half-gallon mason jar to make the tea, I typically have about 1" of dried herbs in the bottom of the jar. Cover the herbs with almost-boiling water and cap tightly. Steep this mixture from four to eight hours. Pour the mixture through a strainer and discard the herbs. The tea will stay fresh for up to five days in the refrigerator.

A small amount of fruit juice (try grape, apple, raspberry) can be added as a sweetener if you like. If the taste is overpowering, then use less herbs and/or brew for a shorter time. If you really don't like the taste, you can try one herb at a time in an attempt to identify the offending taste. Some folks like the Nettles but not the Red Raspberry leaves while for others, it's the other way around. Play with it a bit, till you find a mixture that suits you.

## Purchasing the Herbs

Herbs should be organic or wild-crafted and fresh (dried is fine, but no more than one year old). If the packaging doesn't say "organic" or "wild-crafted," it isn't. Organic, packaged Pregnancy Tea in tea bags is now widely available. It is certainly okay, but not quite the same as what we are recommending here. The amount of herb in the tea bag and the typical length of time that one brews a cup of tea (5 minutes?) will yield an infusion with nowhere near the nutritional content discussed above. You could increase the number of tea bags used and the length of brewing time, but this is not a cost-effective method and likely is not going to deliver the same nutritional boost.

Dried herbs have a shelf life of one year. After that time, the essential oils in the herbs become inactive. A brew made with older herbs may have a funky flavor and the tea will appear cloudy and unappealing. Make sure that your supplier doesn't sell herbs that have been sitting on the shelf for a long time. Mail order is an excellent way to assure both quality and freshness (see recommended sources below) and is also the most cost effective! If you have these plants growing around you, try harvesting them yourself. Put them on a screen to dry, and then store them (even more cost effective).

All herbs should be stored in air-tight containers, in a cool, dark place. Exposure to sunlight and temperature extremes (such as above the stove) will age your herbs more quickly.

## Sources

- **Center for the Childbearing Year.** We sell high-quality, organic tea herbs by the quarter pound and pre-mixed individual Postpartum Herbal Baths. Prices are much lower than those charged by local health food stores, but higher than the cost of ordering by the pound through the mail. We do not mail herbs; they are only available for purchase on site.
- Starwest Botanicals, www.starwest-botanicals.com (has the best prices I have found)
- Mountain Rose Herbs, www.mountainroseherbs.com
- Blessed Herbs, www.blessedherbs.com

## For More Information ...

on the safe use of herbs during pregnancy, labor and birth, and postpartum for both mom and baby, see:

- Susun Weed's book, *Wise Woman Herbal for the Childbearing Year*
- Aviva Romm is an OB/GYN herbalist who provides up-to-date evidence-based information about the safe use of herbs on her website. She has a great blog too. www.avivaromm.com.

# Optimizing Your Prenatal Nutrition

## Increase Fluids
your body weight divided by 2 = # of fluid ounces per day

## Protein
frequent, throughout day, to appetite
(approximately 60-80 grams per day)

## Grains
4-6 servings

## Fresh Fruits
2-4 servings

## Fresh Veggies
3-5 servings

## Fats
do not restrict; eat the good ones!

**Good Fluid Choices:** water, Pregnancy Tea, herbal tea, 100% fruit juice
**Limit:** coffee, caffeinated tea, pop
**Avoid:** alcohol, diet pop, drinks with high fructose corn syrup

**Good Protein Choices:** red meats, whole turkey breast, chicken, legumes, nuts and seeds, dairy, eggs, tofu, fish and seafood; eat organic if possible; eat high protein snacks
**Limit:** lunch meats and other foods loaded with preservatives
**Avoid:** Fish and seafood high in mercury and other heavy metals (see p. 6)

**Eat High-Quality Fats:** olive oil, coconut oil, flax seed oil, butter, whole milk dairy products, avocados, nuts and seeds, high-fat fish and seafood, lard
**Avoid:** hydrogenated fats, margarine, rancid fats

**Eat a Wide Variety of Fresh Fruits & Veggies:** if not fresh, frozen is next best choice; the deeper the color, the higher the vitamin and mineral content (e.g., dark leafy greens are better than iceberg lettuce); organic if possible
**Limit:** dried fruits and fruit juices—both are high in sugar

**Eat Whole Grains Everyday:** brown rice, oatmeal, millet, buckwheat, whole grain breads, etc.
**Limit:** white flour products (white bread, pasta, pastries, etc.), white rice, high-carb treats with refined white sugar, junk food

**Avoid:** empty calories with artificial ingredients

**Condiments & Such:**
Good dressings: high-quality oils and a variety of vinegars (balsamic, cider vinegar, etc.); or mix fresh lemon juice and olive oil with a bit of Dijon mustard
Good additions: kelp powder, sea salt, apple cider vinegar
Good natural sweeteners: maple syrup, honey, molasses
**Limit:** refined white sugar
**Avoid:** artificial sweeteners in any form (e.g., diet pop)

# Common Discomforts of Pregnancy and Alternatives to Drugs for Relief

The following is a guide to the common discomforts of pregnancy, their causes and cures. As a general rule, aches and pains are reduced by good muscle tone, as there is then less strain on ligaments and joints. Women should keep up some regular form of exercise and practice good body mechanics in standing, sitting, rising, walking, climbing, reaching, lifting, etc. Walking and swimming are excellent, especially if you were not already exercising regularly prior to becoming pregnant. Adequate rest and a well-balanced diet also minimize discomforts.

## Leg Cramps

### Cause
- pressure of uterus on blood vessels, lessening the flow of blood to the legs
- overextension of the foot; occurs with pointing of the toes (e.g., when bedcovers are too heavy, with tightly-made bed, or when exercises are improperly done)
- sudden stretching
- fatigue or chilling
- lack of calcium in diet
- excessive amounts of phosphorus absorbed from milk and milk products, which impede the absorption of calcium

### Relief
- stretch the cramped muscle, improving circulation; stretch should be gentle and constant, not jerky
- for foot cramp, stand on affected foot
- for cramp in calf, straighten the knee, flex the foot, hold, then relax and repeat if necessary
- for cramp in front of thigh, stretch leg backward
- for cramp in buttock, stretch leg forward
- NEVER massage a cramped muscle; it enhances the cramp
- try adding more calcium to your diet; sesame seeds, dark leafy greens, and pregnancy tea are excellent non-dairy sources
- soak in an Epsom Salts bath

## Groin Aches or Pains

### Cause
- poor posture
- standing too long
- pressure of baby
- spasm of round ligaments

**Relief**

- do light effleurage (small circular massage) in groin area, giving a slight lift as hands come upward; do not use pressure on the down stroke
- for relief of sudden spasm, pull up leg on same side as spasm, as if tying a shoe, or lie down on affected side with leg drawn up
- try applying heat via a hot water bottle, heating pad or rice soak; or soak in a hot with Epsom Salts bath

## Ache in Back, Hips, or Thighs

**Cause**

- pressure of baby on small nerves inside of vertebrae and pelvis
- shift in mother's center of gravity with accompanying poor posture; more common in multiparas with poor muscle tone; lax abdominal muscles let uterus fall forward, leading to poor posture for maintenance of balance
- softening effect of hormones on connective tissue of spine and sacroiliac joints

**Relief**

- pelvic rock on all fours
- careful attention to correct posture and body mechanics
- when standing, lift one foot and place it on an object so it is higher than the other foot; or stand with one foot in front of the other and rock back and forth slightly
- try a prenatal yoga class
- firm mattress
- chiropractic adjustment may help if what you are feeling is pain rather than ache or stress, or if the problem is chronic
- sciatica, or shooting pain from the buttock down the leg, may be relieved by elevating the legs in a right angle position against the wall
- take care when driving; use a pillow behind your back; adjust the car seat; stretch often on long rides

**Caution:** Be careful not to classify all backaches as to the same cause. Find the exact location and type of pain. Backache waist-high and to one side may indicate kidney problems. Ache in the middle of a buttock with muscle cramping may be due to a sacroiliac problem. Rhythmic lower back pain could be labor.

## Fingers (tingling, numbness, swelling)

**Cause**

- enlargement of breast tissue high in armpit, resulting in pressure on nerves and blood vessels

**Relief**

- place hands on shoulders and rotate elbows in a circle

### Diaphragm Pressure (cramp or stitch under ribs)

**Cause**
- baby high in abdomen, compressing the diaphragm against the base of the lungs

**Relief**
- lift rib cage by raising arms sideways and upward above the head; stretch

### Dyspnea (shortness of breath)

**Cause**
- baby high in abdomen, compressing the diaphragm against the base of the lungs
- may indicate anemia

**Relief**
- sleep propped up with pillows or spend first ten minutes in bed lying on back with arms extended above head and resting back on the bed
- relief occurs later in the pregnancy when the baby engages, or moves deeper in the pelvis
- if anemia is the problem, increase natural sources of iron in diet (raisins, blackstrap molasses, wheat germ, kelp, apricots, and leafy greens – especially kale, Swiss chard, mustard and turnip greens); drink lots of Pregnancy Tea; Floradix Herbs Plus Iron is a natural iron supplement available at health food stores

### Dizziness, Fainting, Lightheadedness

**Cause**
- vasomotor changes
- pressure of uterus on greater abdominal vessels
- anemia
- hypoglycemia

**Relief**
- avoid sudden changes in posture; after lying down, get up slowly, rolling to one side, then slowly push up to a sitting position using your arms
- follow advice regarding anemia above
- do not skip meals; eat good food frequently
- avoid hot, stuffy rooms

### Heartburn

**Cause**
- enlarged uterus displaces stomach upward

- hormones relax cardiac sphincter of stomach, slow digestion, and allow stomach acids to back up into esophagus
- nervous tension, worry and fatigue intensify problem

**Relief**
- eat several small meals a day instead of three large ones
- avoid greasy or highly-spiced foods and coffee
- if problem is especially bad at night, sleep propped up with pillows; don't lie down right after eating
- avoid over-the-counter remedies, especially baking soda and Alka-Seltzer because of their high sodium content; some antacids contain aluminum which is toxic; others contain poorly-assimilated calcium
- try papaya enzyme tablets, umeboshi plum balls, raw almonds or raw cashews (a few, chewed to a pulp)
- gently massaging the stomach downward may help
- a reflexology (foot massage) treatment may help

## Constipation

**Cause**
- diet poor in fiber
- diminished peristalsis due to pressure of enlarged uterus and the relaxing effect of hormones on the smooth muscles of the intestines
- excess iron from prenatal vitamins which the body can't assimilate; turns the stool black

**Relief**
- drink more fluids, especially in the morning to aid elimination
- increase intake of fiber; have at least two servings of whole grains (real oatmeal, brown rice, millet, barley, etc.) daily and increase your intake of fresh, raw fruits and vegetables
- make sure diet contains plenty of B vitamins found in wheat germ, whole grains and Brewer's yeast
- walk more
- when sitting on toilet, put feet up on a small stool; relax pelvic floor
- abandon poor-quality vitamins or iron pills and search for iron-rich foods or high quality food-grown vitamins; drink Pregnancy Tea
- if problem persists, consult your midwife for herbal or homeopathic help and then discover a preventive maintenance plan (such as an apple and brown rice each day, or prunes at night, etc.); it is extremely important to not be constipated during pregnancy

## Hemorrhoids (varicose veins of the lower bowel and rectum)

**Cause**
- relaxing effect of progesterone and pressure of heavy uterus on lower part of large bowel
- obesity
- lack of exercise, excessive sitting
- constipation
- straining to move bowels

**Relief**
- same as for constipation
- do pelvic floor exercises (kegels) regularly to simulate circulation in the pelvic area
- apply cold compresses (e.g., ice, witch hazel)
  Pregnancy Tea to tone the vascular system

## Varicose Veins

**Cause**
- hereditary predisposition
- relaxing effect of progesterone on walls of veins
- pressure of enlarged uterus on abdominal veins slows blood return from lower limbs, so blood tends to pool in the weakened veins
- fatigue
- standing with knees locked, causing muscular constriction which prevents proper venous return
- standing or sitting in one position for a long period of time

**Relief**
- avoid round garters, thigh highs, or any clothing that causes constriction and pressure on any part of the body
- change positions frequently; avoid long standing or sitting without relief
- take walks regularly; the massaging action of muscles close to veins is good for stimulating circulation
- elevate legs several times a day; the more severe the problem, the more frequent the elevation; lie on floor with legs straight up the wall as though sitting on the wall; relax for a few minutes
- wear support hose or stockings made of elastic; put on while lying down, ideally before getting up in the morning
- never stand "at attention" with knees locked; they should always be slightly flexed
- Vitamin E capsules may aid circulation and bring some relief (do not exceed 600 IU per day)
- drink Pregnancy Tea; add Rose Hips for the bioflavonoids

- rutin, a part of the vitamin C complex, can be taken in capsule form, after the first trimester
- for varicosities of the vulva, lie with hips elevated several times a day

**For More Information**

See Susun Weed's book, *Wise Woman Herbal for the Childbearing Year* or Aviva Jill Romm's *Natural Pregnancy Book*. Both are good self-help manuals with reliable information.

# Choosing Your Support Team:  Quiz for Partners

A very important ingredient in your birth support team is your choice of caregiver (midwife or doctor) and place of birth (hospital, birth center, or home). If you are still in the process of choosing a caregiver and a location for your birth, then our free online class, Choices in Childbirth: A Consumer's Guide [www.center4cby.com] is designed to aid you in making an informed decision.

Assuming you have already chosen a caregiver and know where you plan to give birth, I would just like to add that it is your right to feel comfortable with your choice. If you have doubts about your care provider or have considered switching to another provider/setting, it may not be too late to do so (even at the very last minute). Here's a hint: If you find yourself coming home from prenatal visits in tears, then something is off. See if opening lines of communication can provide clarity or resolve any issues. It does not get easier to raise your concerns in labor; they are best addressed prenatally, in a forthright manner. You have a right to feel supported in your choices. You are the consumer here and, one way or another, you are paying the bill.

## Goals for This Exercise

- Moms: (1) Try to anticipate the types of support that you will respond to and (2) understand that your partner may not be the best person to meet ALL of your needs in labor.

- Dads/Partners: (1) Understand the type of support that your partner may require in labor and (2) consider what your role at the birth will be.

- Establish good communication regarding mutual expectations and problem solve any issues *before* the birth (e.g., before an unwanted mother-in-law shows up).

- Plan for success: Give the mother permission to get her needs met in labor. Trust me, this is MUCH better than having unarticulated needs, making assumptions that your partner will meet them, and then being disappointed or resentful when un-communicated needs don't get met. Needs don't go away when we don't honor them; in fact, they often get stronger!

- *Remember, whatever is best for mom is also best for baby.* Your birth is about you and your family. It is okay to ask family and friends to respect your wishes.

## How to Do This Exercise

- Each partner fills out their section of the quiz.

- Next, find a time to share your questions and answers with each other.

- Explore any topics where you might have mismatched expectations or where one person's needs are not a good fit for the partner's ability to fulfill that need. Just identify points of potential conflict, *without judging them.*

- Next, come up with positive solutions for identified challenges. This might involve exploring, for example, hiring a doula. It may be reassuring to know that most doulas offer a no-obligation interview with prospective clients to discover whether the doula and the couple are a good match. If you are wondering about it, go ahead and interview a couple of doulas.

## Questions for the Expectant Mother ~ Worksheet

When feeling stressed, anxious, unwell, or in pain, what do you do to make yourself feel better?

What types of activity help you to relax? (warm bath, music, massage, dark, quiet room, specific activities? other?). List everything that has worked in the past for you.

When others have helped you through a challenging experience, what have they done (specifically) that was helpful? Was there anything that was not helpful, or perhaps even made the challenge more difficult for you (even if it was well intentioned)?

What are your expectations of your partner during your upcoming labor and birth?

Rate each of the following according to the extent you find it comforting.

| | Very comforting | Somewhat helpful | Unsure | Probably not helpful | Definitely not comforting |
|---|---|---|---|---|---|
| Company of others | | | | | |
| To be left alone | | | | | |
| Focused attention | | | | | |
| Reassurance | | | | | |
| Suggestions | | | | | |
| Massage, touch | | | | | |
| Just to be there | | | | | |

**Make a list** of the people in your life who meet the following criteria:
- Would be an asset during the labor and birth process (make it easier on me)
- Share similar beliefs about birth
- Can provide unconditional, nonjudgmental, non-inhibiting support
- Have confidence in me and my capacities
- Are not afraid of birth
- Will be able to witness me in pain without becoming overly upset
- Possess a personality and style capable of meeting my needs in labor, especially helping me to relax
- Are available to be present at my baby's birth
- Want to be present at my baby's birth

Now, identify the person(s) on the list who can also best complement your partner's capacities, limitations and preferences.

Who do you feel would be your ideal support team?

## Questions for the Partner ~ Worksheet

How active a participant in the labor and birth process do you anticipate being? Put a check after each item below that best describes your preferred role.

- Primary support person

- Part of a team providing support

- Witness to birth and emotional support only

- Very hands-on, help with positioning, massage, comfort measures

- Help in making all decisions

- Would like to help catch the baby, cut the umbilical cord

- Want to take a back row seat; view the birth from the mother's perspective

- Would feel disappointed if there wasn't much for me to do to help

- It would be okay with me if I wasn't very involved with hands-on support

- I would prefer to not be present for the birth

- Unsure about my role; want to see how it goes

Is there anything your partner could do in labor that would frighten or upset you?

Are you aware of any expectations regarding your role at the birth that make you feel uncomfortable?

Are there any individuals whom you feel strongly should *not* be present at your baby's birth?

Describe your ideal birth support team.

# What is a Doula? A Consumer's Guide
## to Getting the Help You Need

### What is a doula?

A doula is a labor support professional who "mothers the mother" during childbirth, as well as during the prenatal and postpartum periods. Birth doulas provide support to pregnant women prenatally, through labor and birth, and in the early days postpartum. Postpartum doulas provide in-home services to families, typically lasting from three weeks to three months, or longer with special circumstances. Some doulas combine the birth and postpartum roles into a complete service package, thereby offering continuity of care throughout the childbearing year.

Doulas are non-medical care providers. Their role is limited to informational, emotional, physical and logistical support. They do not provide clinical care such as taking blood pressure or checking dilation in labor, nor do they give medical advice. A "doula" who offers vaginal checks at home in early labor, for example, may be offering a service that you find desirable, however her role is more accurately described as "monitrice" (a clinical role which falls somewhere in between the doula and the midwife role). Postpartum doulas are not "baby nurses," but a nurse may offer in-home care to postpartum families. Likewise, a "doula" who "prescribes" homeopathic or herbal treatments to support healing also may be offering a service that you value, but she is operating outside of the scope of practice of the doula professional.

All doulas provide information, emotional support and comfort measures such as massage, hydrotherapy and enhanced relaxation. Doulas enjoy providing attention to expectant parents and getting to know their clients prenatally. By the time you go into labor, your doula has become a trusted friend and mentor. During labor and birth, doulas feel privileged to be present and helping at such a sacred and joyful event. Postpartum doulas simply love hanging out with new moms and their babies! Your doula is there to support you in your choices and to provide concrete physical and logistical support. Doulas do not take the place of dads, partners or other family members who want to help you. Their job is to facilitate everyone's optimal participation at your birth, as well as to provide support to the entire family through the postpartum recovery and adjustment period. If you are a single mother, your doula can serve as your primary support person so that you are never left alone in labor.

### A selection of services provided by birth doulas:
- Nutritional counseling
- Tips for coping with discomforts of pregnancy
- Preparation for birth
- Assistance in creating a birth plan
- Support at home in early labor
- Comfort measures in labor
- Massage
- Suggestions and support for positioning in labor

- Continuous support throughout labor and birth
- Troubleshooting for difficult births
- Facilitate communication and informed decision making with your health care providers
- Support for dads and partners
- Natural birth coach and advocate
- Support for VBAC (Vaginal Birth After Cesarean)
- Cesarean and post-cesarean support
- Support for the bond between mom and baby in those tender early hours
- Encouragement and skilled support to breastfeed
- Postpartum home visit(s)
- Community resources and referrals

## A selection of services provided by postpartum doulas:
- Breastfeeding support
- Newborn care
- Comfort measures and support for the mother's physical recovery
- Shopping, errands, meal preparation
- Laundry, light cleaning, household organization (not housecleaning)
- Sibling adjustment support (not babysitting or nanny services)
- Depression screening and referrals
- Education on infant topics
- Community resources and referrals

Shifts worked by postpartum doulas vary. Some may do overnights; others may stick to the weekday hours when their children are in school, and so on. Expect a typical shift to be from three to four hours, though some doulas may work an eight-hour day. There are no rule—it is up to you and your doula. Typically, support is more concentrated in the first two weeks and then gradually the family weans off of doula support. However, in special circumstances such as multiples, preemies, babies with special needs, or moms suffering from postpartum depression, postpartum doulas may be involved over a longer period of time with the family

Before hiring a postpartum doula, consider whether or not you are really seeking a nanny for your other children or house cleaning help. If those are your primary motivations, then you should hire a nanny or house cleaner and will probably come out better financially by doing so. Another option may be to start out with a doula for the first couple of weeks while mom is recovering physically, adjusting emotionally, and may be in need of breastfeeding support, and then transition towards hiring a nanny later (say, in the case of twins or multiples).

## What is a certified doula?
A certified doula has chosen to complete a certification process through a doula or childbirth association such as DONA International, CAPPA or others. While certification processes differ, certification generally means that a person has: (1) completed a proscribed training program, (2) documented a minimum level of hands-on experience with positive client evaluations, (3)

completed reading requirements and (4) agreed to work within the Scope of Practice as defined by the certifying organization.

## What do doulas charge for their services?

Because individual doulas are self-employed and set their own rates, there is no precise standard to determine how much you should pay for doula services. Some doulas have a set fee, while others may use a sliding scale so that they can provide services to clients at a range of income levels. Expect doula rates to vary based on level of experience, additional services provided, geographic area and certification status.

In general, birth doulas charge from $600 to $1200 for a package of services that includes the birth. Keep in mind that this fee generally includes phone consultations and prenatal and postpartum visits, as well as compensating the doula for the days and weeks she commits to being on-call for you, in addition to paying for her services at the birth itself. Postpartum doulas generally charge from $20 to $35 per hour. Presumably, the more experienced, and therefore more skilled, doulas are the ones charging the higher fees, with less experienced doulas starting out at the lower end of the scale.

## What are the benefits of doula support?

There have now been several studies on the benefits of continuous labor support on labor and birth outcomes. Laboring women who are supported by doulas have lower c-section rates, lower instrumental delivery (forceps and vacuum extraction) rates and are less likely to use epidurals or pain medication than women who do not have doula support. These women also have shorter labors, have more positive childbirth experiences overall and are more likely to breastfeed. Furthermore, the newborns of women receiving doula support have higher one-minute and five-minute Apgar scores (a routine assessment of the newborn's well-being immediately post-birth).

Postpartum doulas can have a strong impact on early parenting success. The evidence shows that women who use a postpartum doula have increased rates of breastfeeding, decreased rates of postpartum depression, a stronger bond with their newborns, greater self-confidence in their parenting abilities and increased understanding of newborn care.

## Is it appropriate to have a doula if my partner will be at the birth?

Yes! The doula's role includes supporting the laboring woman and her partner. Your doula should be able to work alongside your partner and/or other family members and show him/her/them how to best support you. If you and your partner have taken childbirth classes, the doula can remind you of techniques you learned in class and provide guidance through the physical and emotional challenges of labor and birth. Your doula can enable your partner to take a break, facilitate communication with your care providers and, in short, be an excellent addition to your birth team.

## Is a doula appropriate if I have an epidural?

Yes! Many women are unsure of whether they will want an epidural (or know they will want one) prior to going into labor. While you should ask your doula if she is comfortable working with women who choose a medicated birth, the role of the doula is not to critique your birth choices but rather to support you and ensure that your wishes are respected. A doula can improve your chances of having an unmedicated birth if that is what you prefer, but she should also be able to provide you with non-judgmental emotional and physical support in the context of a medicated birth. Women who choose to use an epidural during labor can especially benefit from a doula during the pushing stage, as this stage can take longer for medicated births due to the decreased physical sensations intrinsic to the use of epidurals. In addition, because the medications used often make babies less alert than normal, it is extremely helpful to have a doula during the immediate postpartum period so that she can support early breastfeeding efforts. Epidurals provide pain relief, not emotional support!

## Is a doula appropriate if I am having a planned cesarean birth?

Yes! Although women having planned cesareans do not experience labor in the same way as women planning vaginal births, a doula can still be helpful to prepare you for the experience. Your doula can help you learn about the choices that you have in the context of a cesarean birth and can also provide emotional support before, during and after the surgery. Because recovery from a cesarean often takes longer and is more complex than recovery from a vaginal birth, a doula can be an asset to parents during the postpartum period. A postpartum doula can help with newborn care, provide breastfeeding support, prepare meals and help take care of your home while you recover from surgery.

## Tips on hiring a doula

- First, screen to see who is accepting clients around your due date.

- Ask how much the doula charges and what services are included in her fee.

- If the answers to the first two questions lead you to want to pursue the possibility of hiring this person, then you could ask for some time for a short phone interview.

- Ask about her level of experience, whether or not she has been formally trained as a doula, whether or not she is certified, and what her philosophy of care is (e.g., what are her thoughts and experience with breastfeeding?). You might want to know if she is a mother herself, what she thinks her biggest strength as a doula is, what she enjoys most about her work, etc. For a more complete list of questions, see below.

- An enthusiastic but inexperienced doula with whom you feel a warm rapport may be preferable to a more experienced doula with whom you feel uncomfortable, for any reason. The best way to choose your doula is to consider the fact that the doula will be present at your birth, or providing in-home support at a time when you may feel vulnerable. Ask yourself with whom you (and your partner) feel the most comfortable. Just what are you looking for? What helps you when you are feeling stressed?

Information, humor, kindness, massage, a flexible attitude, a good listener? Are you looking for a mother figure or more of a big sister? The personality and beliefs of your doula may well be more important than any other factor. If you choose to interview one or more doulas, it can be helpful to ask the following questions. In the final decision, trust your gut. A less experienced, uncertified doula may resonate better with you than the most experienced doula in town. This is only about getting your needs met.

- As you move through this process, you can narrow down your selection to one or two people with whom you and your partner (if any) would like to meet in person for a more in-depth interview.

- Ask for and check references. The most useless doula in the world is the one who is unreliable (if she doesn't answer her phone when you are in labor, who cares how skillful or "nice" she is?). Doulas who have created good word-of-mouth about their services are likely to endeavor to ensure that you too are a satisfied customer.

- Check credentials. If the doula claims to be a DONA International-certified doula, you can confirm her certification online by checking with her professional organization.

- Does the doula have an agenda (my way or the highway)? If so, is her agenda congruent with yours? Try to think of a few questions before the interview that are designed to get at the answers most important to you. Have your partner articulate any questions or concerns he/she may have as well. In the end, make sure you hire someone who can provide non-judgmental support for you and your family. You don't want to have to hide your diet pop cans or your toddler's play guns when your doula comes to your home, nor apologize for a medicated birth if those are your choices. (I'm having a hard time letting the diet pop statement stand, because it's SO bad for you, but I hope that makes my point about non-judgmental support … I would not be the doula for you if you wanted me to bring you your diet pop in labor, or at least, I would be very challenged in this regard.)

- In the case of hiring a postpartum doula, many couples find themselves in a rather urgent frame of mind ("Can you start today?"). Consider starting with a one-week commitment from your doula with the possibility of extending beyond that time frame. If integrating a stranger into your home proves more stressful than helpful, you may have chosen the wrong doula.

## Sample questions to ask a prospective doula
- How long have you been in practice as a doula?

- How many families have you served?

- What training have you completed to prepare you for this role?

- Are you certified?

- What is your philosophy about your doula work and its purpose?

- Are you a mother yourself? (This may or may not be important to you. Doulas who are not mothers themselves may have more time to focus on you and your needs, while doulas who are mothers themselves certainly will bring an added dimension of understanding to their care. On the other hand, experienced mothers may be more opinionated about the "right" way to do things, based upon their own beliefs and experiences. Look for someone capable of flexible, non-judgmental support or, if she has an agenda, make sure it's the same as yours!)

- Do you have experience with other clients whose situations are similar to mine (e.g., first-time mothers, natural vs. medicated birth, same hospital, home births, older mothers, single mothers, VBAC moms, etc.)?

- How much do you charge? What is included in your fee (prenatal/postnatal visits, phone support)? Do you require payment up front? What is your refund policy?

- Do you work with a backup doula?

- Do you have any references from families with whom you have worked?

**Additional questions for birth doulas**
- How certain are you that you will be able to attend my birth? Do you have any other commitments during that time period?

- How do you picture yourself supporting me and my partner during the birth?

- Do you provide labor support at home in early labor for women planning hospital deliveries?

- Do you only work as a birth doula or can we also hire you for postpartum work if needed?

**Additional questions for postpartum doulas**
- Are you available for overnight help, weekend help, daytime help, etc.?

- How much experience do you have providing breastfeeding support?

- What services do you provide or exclude? (For example, some doulas may be willing to do some sibling care, scrub out a bath tub, or walk the dog, while others may not. Really think through what it is that you need and then ask questions to determine if the doula can meet your needs.)

- Do you have any add-on services (such as bringing meals, massage, etc.)?

# Prenatal Perineal Massage

There is no hard evidence that prenatal perineal massage is linked with better birth outcomes or, more specifically, lowering the incidence of trauma to the perineum. However, there is a growing body of anecdotal evidence that the practice of perineal massage is helpful. Midwives report that women who practice perineal massage regularly in the last six weeks of pregnancy experience less stinging sensation during crowning and are less likely to tear or get an episiotomy. An added value is that the practice familiarizes a woman with stretching sensations in this area so she will more easily relax these muscles when stinging occurs just before the moment of birth.

Several other factors will influence whether or not a woman tears or experiences an episiotomy at her birth including:

- Choice of caregiver
- Decision to have an epidural (increases risk)
- Consent to vacuum or forceps (some degree of trauma is a certainty)
- Maternal position at delivery (best to use a position that equalizes the pressure of the head coming through the tissues)
- Physiologic, spontaneous pushing efforts versus coached pushing
- Skill of caregiver in preventive techniques and the art of gentle vaginal birth
- Baby's tolerance of second stage
- Health of maternal tissues (nutritional status; absence/presence of various vaginal infections with discharge that irritates the tissues)
- Past trauma, sexual abuse, or assault leading to fear and tension in the mother

In conclusion, prenatal perineal massage may help promote the development of a healthy mind/body connection that women can tap into at birth. There is no evidence that neglecting the practice altogether puts women at risk for tearing. So feel free to take a playful approach; it can only help.

## Directions

- The massage can be done with a partner or by the woman alone.

- Wash your hands and trim your nails. Sit in a warm, comfortable area, spreading your legs apart in a semi-sitting birthing position. To become familiar with your perineal area, use a mirror for the first couple of massages (a floor-to-ceiling mirror works best). Use massage oil, such as pure vegetable oil, olive oil, calendula oil, etc. Avoid petroleum-based oil, such as Vaseline as it disrupts the normal vaginal flora. Apply the oil to your fingers and thumbs and around your perineum.

- Insert your thumbs as deeply as you can inside your vagina. Press the perineal area down toward the rectum and toward the sides. Gently continue to stretch this opening until you feel a slight burn or tingling.

- Hold this stretch until the tingling subsides and gently massage the lower part of the vaginal canal back and forth.

- While massaging, hook your thumbs onto the sides of the vaginal canal and gently pull these tissues forward, as your baby's head will do during delivery.

- Finally, massage the tissues between the thumb and forefinger, back and forth, for about a minute.

- Being too vigorous could cause bruising or swelling in these sensitive tissues or tension in the muscles—all counterproductive! If the massage is experienced as painful, back off, slow down and honor your feelings.

- During the massage, avoid pressure on the urethra as this could induce irritation in that area. Think of the perineum as the face of a clock. If you were looking at it from the partner's perspective, focus the massage between 10 and 2, or the lower two-thirds of the opening.

- As you become more comfortable with this process, try integrating kegel exercises into the routine to help you get the feel for your pelvic floor muscles.

- Frequency? As you wish—anywhere from daily starting at 36 weeks to a frequency of your own desire. Perhaps 3–4 times per week for 5–15 minutes?

*CAUTION: **Do not do perineal massage if the bag of waters is broken or in the presence of an active herpes outbreak or other vaginal infection.***

# Homeopathic Preparation for Delivery

If you are inclined towards complementary medicine, then you may be interested to know that many homeopaths recommend the following remedies be taken during the last month of pregnancy to help prepare the woman for labor. Follow your instincts and, if homeopathy is not normally a method of health care that you use—and therefore you do not already understand or have a degree of confidence in how it works—then, by all means, feel free to skip this recommendation. Certainly, every woman does not require that preventive measures be taken, but there are some who may benefit. I particularly encourage first-time mothers and women who have a history of post-dates pregnancies, dysfunctional labors with failure to progress, or unusually long labors to give the regimen a try.

### Caulophyllum 30C (Blue Cohosh)
Blue Cohosh is a natural source of oxytocin (the hormone that causes the uterus to contract). It helps produce effective contractions and is used to initiate or enhance labor. When homeopathically prepared, it will not bring on contractions if the woman is not ready to go into labor and, indeed, may relieve excessive toning (a.k.a. "Braxton-Hicks") contractions.

### Cimicifuga 30C (Black Cohosh)
To ease fear of giving birth. Cimicifuga complements the action of Caulophyllum by aiding the uterus to contract in a coordinated and effective way. Cimicifuga also works to relieve displaced labor pains such as sciatica, hip cramps and the like.

### Arnica 30C
To avoid the physical trauma which may be associated with childbirth. Arnica can prevent excess blood loss, shock and trauma to soft tissues. It is often used prophylactically prior to surgery, dental treatments and so on. After the birth, both mom and baby can be given repeated doses if any swelling, bruising or pain are experienced. Arnica speeds the healing process.

### Directions
Start taking the remedies four weeks prior to your due date. Take each remedy once per week, alternating as follows: Caulophyllum on Monday, Cimicifuga on Wednesday, and Arnica on Friday.

Homeopathic remedies should be taken by tapping the correct dosage into the bottle cap and then tapping the pellets into your mouth, being careful not to handle the pellets directly or get saliva on the bottle cap. The number of pellets equaling one dose depends upon the size of the pellets (10–15 poppy-seed-size and 2–3 of the larger variety). Remedies should be administered into a clean mouth with nothing to eat or drink 15 minutes before and after the remedy is given.

Essential oils and aromatic oils such as mints, camphor, menthol and oils found in coffee should be avoided altogether during the weeks when you are taking homeopathics as these substances tend to render the remedies ineffective.

# Optimal Fetal Positioning

## What is Optimal Fetal Positioning?

"Optimal Fetal Positioning" is the term used to describe the best possible position for your baby to be in prior to birth. The optimal position is when your baby lays head down, facing your back, with your baby's back on either side of your belly button. This is known as **"occiput anterior."**

Having your baby in the occiput anterior position makes for an easier birth. In that position, your baby is best lined up to pass through your pelvis. Your baby's head is flexed with his chin tucked into his chest, which means the smallest part of his head is presenting first and he can more easily maneuver his way through your pelvis.

Conversely, when babies engage in the pelvis in the **"occiput posterior" position** (baby's back lying along mom's spine and facing her belly), this typically results in a dysfunctional labor pattern with greatly increased pain, often centered in the back. Common features of a posterior labor are:

- Slow progress, often stalled completely at 5 or 6 cm dilation
- Asymmetrical dilation of the cervix, due to the baby's head not fitting well into the bony pelvis and consequently not evenly applied to the cervix
- Low back pain, often intense; may be somewhat neutralized by counter pressure on the sacrum
- Back pain that does not go away altogether between contractions

If mom does reach complete dilation with a posterior-presenting baby, it often takes a tremendous effort to push out a baby in this position. Many cesareans are done for lack of progress, in either first or second stage of labor, due to this cause.

In the case of a baby presenting in the **breech position** (butt, knees, or feet coming first), current practice dictates cesarean delivery. Approximately 3 percent of babies will be breech at term. While vaginal breech delivery for certain specific breech presentations can be safe, overall, there is a higher incidence of complications in vaginal breech deliveries. The current generation of doctors has not been trained in handling the complicated breech; that knowledge has been retained by a few old-timers and the homebirth midwives. Ironically, some women are choosing to have homebirths with their breech babies as their only option to surgical delivery. Since the risks are higher with both posterior and breech presentations, certainly it makes sense to do everything in our power to encourage babies into the optimal fetal position.

## How Can You Avoid a Posterior Baby?

First off, if it's not broke, you don't need to fix it and you can relax! Try to "tune in" to your baby's position prenatally. At prenatal visits after 30 weeks gestation, most care providers begin to put hands on your belly during a prenatal visit to determine the baby's size and position in the pelvis. Old-time doctors and most midwives are familiar with "the art of palpation" and have developed this skill. Many of the younger generation of doctors (and some medicalized midwives) have become overly reliant on ultrasound for the "window into the womb" that it provides and have not mastered this skill. They may not believe it is important to determine the baby's position unless they suspect a breech presentation.

If your care provider IS putting hands on, engage them in a conversation about what they are feeling. Ask them if they know where the baby's back is. If, at 30 weeks, your baby is determined to be in a breech or posterior position, then just make a note of it. Typically, at this point in the pregnancy, the baby is still floating well above the pubic bone and there is plenty of room to turn. If, at subsequent prenatals, the baby has adopted a different position, then that is simply a sign that there is plenty of room and the baby is still moving. However, if your baby shows a pattern of preferring a breech or posterior position, and he/she has not moved out of that position by approximately 36 weeks, then it may be time to get proactive and do what you can to encourage the baby to turn and adopt a more favorable position for birth.

There are things you can do to improve your chances of having your baby lie in an occiput anterior position. The back of your baby's head and his back are the heaviest body parts. By keeping your body posture in an upright or slightly forward position, you can help keep those heaviest parts of your baby pointing down, facing your back, with his back on either side of your belly button, in the optimal position.

Below are some ideas to keep in mind during the last few weeks of your pregnancy, to help your baby engage in the optimal position:

- Mentally draw a line starting from your back through your body and out through your belly button. Try to consistently sit and stand in a position where that line would be either completely level or pointing downwards.

- Positions to limit or avoid are:
  o Sitting in chairs that have you leaning back (i.e., recliner chairs, bucket car seats, etc.). Placing a foam wedge on your car seat can help keep your posture straight in bucket car seats.
  o Crossing your legs; this reduces the space in front of your pelvic where you want your baby to be, while opening up the space at the back of your pelvis.
  o Lying on your back to sleep.

- Positions to encourage are:
  o Sitting on a birth ball
  o Straddling a kitchen chair backwards
  o Sitting in any position that keeps your knees lower than your hips
  o Walking
  o Swimming with your belly down (i.e., front crawl, breast stroke)
  o Sitting in yoga positions (i.e., tailor position, or with heels together)

54

- Lying on your side to sleep (or, even better, on a ¾ angle leaning towards the bed)
- Adopting a hands-and-knees position and doing "pelvic rocks" several times a day (this position is my favorite, especially for very late pregnancy; try moving to the floor for a few pelvic rocks after each trip to the bathroom)

## Strategies to Turn Breech Babies

- Breech tilt position; mom lies on an inclined plane, with feet elevated and head down at an angle of approximately 30 degrees; rest in this position for approximately 15 minutes; repeat 2–3 times per day until baby turns.

- Moxibustion; technique from Traditional Chinese Medicine involves applying the herb Mugwort (which has been rolled into a compressed cone shape) to an acupuncture point on the baby toe, and lighting it on fire, thereby transferring heat to the point; used in China for centuries to turn breech babies, it has been written up in the American Journal of Obstetrics and Gynecology as being an evidence-based practice; find an acupuncturist or practitioner of Traditional Chinese Medicine in your area who is familiar with the technique.

- External version is offered by some hospitals; technique involves manually forcing the baby to turn to a head-down position; done in conjunction with ultrasound because it sometimes causes fetal distress; waiver for surgery must be signed ahead of time; procedure is widely reported to be painful by mothers.

## Other Techniques/Treatments for Breech and Posterior Presentation

- Webster Technique; chiropractic technique with good success rate
- Visualization; picture your baby in the optimal fetal position
- Homeopathic Pulsatilla and Natrum Muriatricum are two of the most commonly-indicated remedies for encouraging the baby to adopt the optimal fetal position (see p. 53)

## Tune In!

Belly Mapping is a fun way to "tune in" to your baby's position in the womb. Check out Gail Tully's website [www.spinningbabies.com] for instructions on how to "map" your baby's position. Gail has produced *The Belly Mapping Workbook*, with great illustrations and step-by-step instructions.

# Homeopathy to Turn a Baby in an Unfavorable Position

Approximately four weeks before the due date, in conjunction with the usually recommended exercises for breech or posterior presentation, homeopathic intervention may assist the baby in getting into a favorable birthing position. The program can be started earlier than four weeks if the woman is very short-waisted and baby consistently prefers to be breech or posterior, or later if there is plenty of room and baby's position has been changeable. Even in labor, remedies are worth a try, but chances for success are reduced after the bag of waters has broken and/or the presenting part has engaged in the pelvis.

First, determine whether there seems to be a normal amount of amniotic fluid around the baby. Too much fluid will keep the baby buoyant and the uterus overextended, so the baby can just float into an undesirable position. Too little fluid will likewise be problematic as the breech baby will not have enough buoyancy to turn. If fluid levels seem to be off in either direction, try the water-balancing tissue salt **Natrum Muriaticum.** Suggested regimens for varying potencies are as follows:

> 6X 3 times per day for 1 week or
> 30C 2 times per day for 3 days or
> 200C once per day for 3 days

Choice of potency may depend on what is available to you and how much time you have to work with this problem. Discontinue any dosing if you don't get results or once the baby has turned.

Now, if fluid levels feel normal, then **Pulsatilla** is the remedy of choice and the one that has the longest reputation in the homeopathic literature for turning babies. According to Farrington (in his Clinical Materia Medica), Pulsatilla acts on the muscular walls of the uterus and stimulates their growth. Sometimes the uterus develops more on one side than another during pregnancy, and with this irregularity, the baby assumes an irregular position. Pulsatilla may alter this uneven growth and permit the baby to assume the proper position. (Follow same dosage recommendations as above.)

If the woman does not fit the overall Pulsatilla or Natrum Muriaticum symptom pictures, or the baby needs to remain in his/her present position for whatever reason, the remedy may not work. If it does work, it is a most gentle intervention indeed, effecting changes in the baby's environment rather than impacting the baby directly.

**For More Information**

*Guide to Homeopathic Remedies for the Birth Bag, 5th Edition,* by Patty Brennan (available at www.center4cby.com]

# Baby Stuff: What Do You Really Need?

**Bedding, Towels**
- Baby towels & washcloths (not necessary; regular towels work just fine; hooded baby towels are nice)
- Bumper pads, pillow, blanket, comforter (no longer considered safe; not recommended)
- Fitted mattress cover and crib sheet (an extra set would be convenient)

**Clothing\***
- Overall, used infant clothing is abundantly available at significant savings; infants grow out of their clothes before they wear them out; just check for stains on used clothing.
- A newborn might go through three or more outfits in one day. You can figure on needing to do a load of laundry every three days or so.
- Pick items that are easy to take on and off; onesies are fine, but it's nice to have some two-piece outfits as well (then you only have to change the half that needs it).
- A couple of cotton hats
- Socks

**Diaper Options (choose one or try a combination approach)\***
- Cloth diapers, diaper covers, diaper pail or
- Diaper service (pick up and deliver once a week; service provides the diaper pail) or
- Disposables (buy newborn size)
- Diaper wipes (convenient, but water and a cloth works)
- Diaper bag or backpack*

**Equipment**
- Baby monitor (convenient but not necessary)
- Bottle warmer (not necessary for breastfeeding moms)
- Electric breast pump (for breastfeeding moms who need to leave baby for hours at a time; basic pump plus accessories which must be sized for the mother; storage bags/bottles)*
- High chair (won't be needed for a few months)*
- Infant car seat*
- Stroller (most folks appreciate this option, though some devoted baby wearers find strollers to be superfluous)

**Furniture**
- Bassinet (baby typically grows out of this by about three months; not necessary)
- Bouncy seat (not necessary)
- Crib & crib mattress (unless you are committed to co-sleeping; might still be a good option for naps)
- Changing table or changing pad for top of existing dresser (convenient and can double as storage for clothing, but not necessary)

- Dresser (not necessary)
- Rocking chair (nice, but babies like to be bounced on a birth ball as well; be sure arm height of chair is not too high for nursing baby)
- Wind-up swing (not necessary; if someone gives/loans you one, you can give it a try; not useful past 3 months)

**Miscellaneous**
- Baby bath (a variety of devices are on the market; convenient, but not necessary; a towel-lined sink works too)
- Mirror for back seat of car so driver can see baby's face*
- Nursing pillow (not necessary, see if you feel you need one)
- Pacifiers (not recommended for at least the first three weeks, until milk supply is well established; may be habit forming)
- Pack n' Play (convenient for overnights)
- Personal care items such as baby shampoo, soap and cream (buy natural baby care items if possible; usually calendula based, which is gentle for the skin); baby comb & hair brush*
- Receiving blankets (at least 3; some larger-size blankets are nice)*
- Shade for car window next to baby*
- Sling or baby carrier (lots of brands and styles on the market)*
- White noise machine (not necessary)

**The following items should NOT be previously owned:**
- Breast pump
- Car seat (unless you know the history; if a car seat has been involved in an accident, it is no longer trustworthy)
- Crib mattress, or ill-fitting mattress for crib (danger of SIDS)

\* These items are needed.

# Labor & Birth Topics

# The Process of Labor and Birth
## Summary Sheet

## Pre-Labor Changes

### Changes in Late Pregnancy (last four weeks or so)
- Baby engages ("drops") in the pelvis. For first-time mothers, this typically happens approximately two weeks prior to birth, though it can be weeks prior or even wait until labor has begun. For a second or more baby, engagement can happen any time.
- Mom may feel increased pressure on her bladder; pressure on diaphragm is relieved; sometimes pubic bone feels sore.
- Emotionally, mom may be feeling discouraged, anxious, excited, tired of being pregnant, etc.
- Cervix begins to soften, ripen and move forward, typically any time after 36 weeks.
- Cervix may begin to efface (thin) and dilate (open).

### Signs of Impending Labor (one day or two prior to onset of labor)
- Frequent, loose bowel movements (may also accompany onset of contractions)
- Nesting instinct with sense of urgency regarding particular chores, errands, purchases that must happen *NOW*. (Note to partners: this is not necessarily a rational process; just go with it.)

## First Stage of Labor (Effacement & Dilation of Cervix)

### Three ways for labor to begin:

1. **Bloody show:** mucus plug dislodges from the cervix; because there are capillaries in the cervix and the cervix is changing, the mucus is likely to be tinged with blood; may or may not be accompanied by noticeable contractions.

2. **Contractions:** the pattern here can be pretty much anything from one per hour lasting 15 seconds, to every 10 minutes, lasting 30 seconds or more; endless variations; may or may not be accompanied by bloody show; contractions may feel like menstrual cramps or may be felt in the low back as an intermittent backache; contractions do not go away when mom changes her position or activity level; most women report that labor contractions feel "different" than the toning contractions of late pregnancy (aka "Braxton-Hicks contractions"). The term "false labor" is used in the instance that a woman experiences contractions that are regular for a time, but disappear altogether when she changes her position or activity level.

3. **Spontaneous Rupture of Membranes (SROM):** bag of water breaks and fluid gushes from the vagina; can also be experienced as a slow leak which may be hard to

differentiate from urine leakage (not terribly uncommon in late pregnancy with weight of baby sitting directly on top of the bladder); care provider can determine the difference with simple office visit to check pH of fluid that is present; expect differences among care providers regarding willingness to wait for labor contractions to begin on their own once SROM has occurred; note whether or not the fluid is clear or has a brownish-green tint to it; if it is not clear, then the baby has passed meconium in utero (the first bowel movement) indicating a need to monitor the baby more closely in labor. SROM is the first sign of labor in about 10 percent of women; it is more typical for the bag of waters to break later in the birth process (>7cm dilation).

### Early Labor
- Cervix continues to ripen, efface, move forward and begins dilating.
- Contractions progress, possibly with bloody show and/or rupture of membranes.
- Contractions get longer and stronger and closer together.
- Mom may feel excited, confident, optimistic, anxious, performance anxiety….
- Mom can talk through contractions and do other activities between contractions.
- Mom may focus more than necessary on the contractions.

### What to do?
- Check the instructions your doctor/midwife/doula has given you regarding when they want to be notified if you think you are in labor and follow those instructions; medical caregiver will advise when it is time to come in; doula may join you at home or at the hospital.
- If membranes are ruptured, do not put anything inside the vagina; be careful about hygiene (keeping bacteria from the rectum away from vaginal opening); refrain from tub baths until you are in active labor.
- An adrenaline rush often accompanies onset of labor; remind mom to save this energy for the hard work that is to come; help her to relax, deep breathing, warm bath if membranes are intact, etc.
- If at night: SLEEP (or at least rest)!
- Eat, drink, empty bladder frequently. VERY IMPORTANT!
- Alternate distracting activities (bath, music, walk, cards, reading, movie, computer games) with rest if tired.
- When contractions become more regular, time them for a while (4 or 5 at a time, every few hours or when labor seems to have changed).

### Active Phase (4–8 cm dilation)
- Cervix is now 100% effaced and 4 cm dilated.
- Contractions continuing to get longer and stronger and closer together, typically coming 3–5 minutes apart and lasting at least 1 minute.
- Mom's attention is increasingly drawn inward; no longer distractible; the labor has become everything—getting through one contraction at a time, recovering and getting ready for the next contraction.

- Mom is working hard; may be sweating and breathing differently; can no longer talk through a contraction; she may be tensing during contractions.
- Cervix continues dilating and baby's head begins to rotate as he/she moves deeper in the pelvis.
- May continue to see bloody show or bag of waters may rupture anytime.
- "Moment of truth;" mom may feel trapped, discouraged, recognizing labor is not within her control.
- May resent disturbances and interruptions.
- May want pain medications. If not, then natural pain management techniques and comfort measures can be used.

### What to do?
- When the shift happens to active labor, you may want to head to the hospital/birth center or have your midwife on her way to you (for homebirth).
- In any case, doula (or other support team members) should join you now.
- Drink fluids and keep bladder empty.
- Help mom with relaxation; begin coping ritual.
- Provide relief with comfort measures.
- "Labor voice," murmuring soothing, encouraging words.

### Transition (8–10 cm)
- Contractions are very close, peak intensity (1–2 minutes apart, lasting approximately 1.5 minutes); contractions may piggyback.
- Mom may vomit.
- Mom may get lost in the intensity of the labor; feel afraid or panicky.
- Mom may scream, thrash, tense, weep, or protest; she is likely to say she "can't go on," "how much longer?" and so on.
- Bloody show may be present or rupture of membranes may occur.
- Mom may start to feel "pushy."

### What to do?
- Move in close, establish eye contact and provide minute-to-minute support.
- Remind her that this is the shortest phase of labor.
- Hang in there!

### The Rest & Be Thankful Phase of Labor (10 cm dilated)
- For some women, labor can slow down at complete dilation.
- This resting phase is often not acknowledged by some care providers who may call for Pitocin or encourage voluntary pushing efforts.
- Mom may experience relief, renewed energy, enthusiasm, hope, or readiness to "get on with it."

### What to do?

- Empty bladder now, before pushing efforts begin.
- Drink, maybe something with a little sweetness to it (cup of hot tea with a generous spoonful of honey).
- Negotiate with care provider regarding letting labor unfold at its own pace.
- Help mom get comfortable, dark room, quiet.
- Rest!

## 2nd Stage of Labor (Descent & Birth of Baby)

### Descent Phase

- Contractions are 3–5 minutes apart and lasting about 1 minute, perhaps a little longer.
- Mom may feel an urge to push with contractions.
- Mom may feel rectal pressure, as though she has to pass a bowel movement.
- Mom may spontaneously hold her breath for part of a contraction or make deep grunting sounds.
- Baby rotates and descends.
- It may take a few contractions for mom to get her new rhythm and feel effective with pushing.
- As baby makes it under the pubic bone, the head may start to be visible at the vaginal opening; a little more with each contraction, but disappearing between contractions.
- Mom may try to pull away from/resist sensation of pressure and stretching as baby moves down.
- Mom may pass stool during this phase, as the baby compresses the lower bowel.
- Nurse or midwife is in the room now, until the birth; if OB is attending, they will likely come in close to the end and L&D nurse will be attending you during most of 2nd stage.
- Caregiver may be doing coached or directed pushing.

### What to do?

- Encourage mom to try different upright positions (especially if progress is slow).
- Keep breathing and use lower (not high-pitched) sounds.
- "Down and out." "Let the baby come."
- If a lot of stool is passing, or mom is especially concerned about it, see if she can do some pushing on the toilet for a while.
- Provide physical support for positioning, if needed.
- Encourage her and give her progress reports; if mom wants to see, set up a mirror for her, or encourage her to reach down and touch her baby's head, or tell her when you can first see the baby's head.
- Keep offering fluids.
- Cool wash cloths to face and neck, between contractions.
- Remind caregiver regarding any points in your Birth Plan related to episiotomy or immediate post-birth care (e.g., delayed cord clamping, skin-to-skin).

### Crowning & Birth

- Head no longer rocks back and forth, but remains visible at vaginal opening, even between contractions.
- Mom feels a burning sensation as baby's head stretches her tissues.
- Caregiver may do episiotomy at this time.
- Caregiver (OB or midwife) is calling the shots at this time.
- As the head emerges, baby rotates and then the shoulders birth one at a time, followed by the rest of the baby's body.
- Baby may be placed directly on mom's belly, with the cord intact (recommended) or the cord may be severed and baby removed to warming table for routine procedures.

### What to do?

- When mom feels "the burn," help her slow down pushing efforts by panting; as long as the breath is going in and out, she is not pushing; establish eye contact if necessary to help her with this; keep the breath in the upper chest.
- Care provider applies a little counter pressure to perineum, oil, hot compresses, if desired.
- Remind doctor/midwife of pertinent requests in Birth Plan (especially regarding episiotomy, cord cutting if requesting delay).

## 3rd Stage (Delivery of the Placenta)

- Contractions continue, though with much less discomfort.
- As the uterus gets smaller and smaller, the placenta no longer has a surface area to be attached to and it is released from the uterine wall, followed by a gush of blood.
- Attendant will encourage mom to push out her placenta.
- Once the placenta has been delivered, the nurse/midwife will periodically check the uterus for firmness, to ensure that it stays contracted in order to shut off blood vessels at the site and control bleeding.
- Baby is either skin-to-skin with mom (recommended) or under heat lamp in container, typically a few feet from the bed.
- Putting baby to breast releases oxytocin, which helps the uterus to contract.

### What to do?

- Continue to advocate for your Birth Plan.
- Allow the baby access to the breast.

## Immediate Postpartum Period (first 2 hours)

- Some moms may get "the shakes."
- Continue bonding/breastfeeding.
- Routine medical procedures for newborn (weighing, Vitamin K, eye prophylaxis, newborn bath).
- Nurse/midwife stays close at hand and monitors mom's bleeding and baby's vital sign.
- Mom helped up to bathroom, to keep bladder empty.

- Mom washed up a bit or an herbal bath is drawn for mom and baby (homebirth, some birth centers).
- Meal for mom and partner.

### What to do?
- Warm mom with blankets.
- Continue to advocate for your Birth Plan (perhaps delaying non-critical newborn procedures for an hour or two).
- Take pictures; make phone calls; receive visitors, if desired.
- Celebrate! Rest.

## Immediate Postpartum Period after Cesarean Delivery
- Mom will go to post-op recovery room with partner. Baby will accompany, provided baby has not been transferred to a Special Care Nursery or the Neonatal Intensive Care Unit (NICU).
- Other visitors may be allowed in at this time.
- If baby is in NICU, dad/partner may want to stay with the baby; doula or other support team member stays with mom until she is stable enough to be brought to baby.
- Mom may have "the shakes." Some women feel nauseated from the anesthesia after surgery. Anti-nausea medications may be given.
- Usually good pain control at this time, from epidural.
- Once stable, mom and baby are moved to a postpartum room; may go back to room you which you were laboring in some hospitals.

### What to do?
- If baby is with you, enjoy your baby, skin-to-skin, near the breast; baby may root and latch on his/her own; just provide access.
- Continue to advocate for any parts of your Birth Plan involving after-birth care.
- If dad/partner is with the baby elsewhere, touch your baby if possible; talk to your baby; call your baby by name; let the baby know you are there.
- If mom and baby are separated, have a support person relay information (and pictures!) of baby to mom; back and forth, until they are together.
- Take pictures, make calls, receive visitors if desired.
- Celebrate! Rest.

# The Three R's: Relaxation, Rhythm and Ritual

There are three characteristics common to women who are observed to be coping well with pain in labor.

1. They are able to **RELAX** during labor and/or between contractions. In early labor, relaxation is a realistic and desirable goal. As labor progresses, many women cope much better if they don't try to relax during contractions. They may feel better if they move or vocalize during the contractions, or even tense parts of their bodies. It is vital, however, that they relax and remain calm between contractions.

2. The use of **RHYTHM** characterizes their coping style. This can be anything from slow dancing with their partner, to leaning over a birth ball and swaying the hips, bouncing on the birth ball, counting out loud, using a rhythmic breathing technique, repeating sounds or words, and so on.

3. They find and use **RITUALS.** The ritual is repeated use of personally meaningful rhythmic activities with every contraction. At first, women may draw heavily on coping measures they learned in childbirth class. However, those who cope well usually do more than that—they discover their own rituals spontaneously in labor. If disturbed in their ritual, or prevented from doing the things they have found to be helpful, laboring women may become upset and stressed.

Women are most likely to find their own coping style when they feel safe and supported, are free from restrictions on their mobility and vocal sounds, and are also free from disturbances to their concentration, such as other people talking to them, or doing procedures on them during contractions. Following are some examples of unplanned, spontaneous rituals discovered by laboring women:

- One woman felt safe and cared for when her mother brushed her long, straight hair rhythmically during the contractions.
- Another rocked in a rocking chair in rhythm with her own pattern of breathing.
- Another wanted her partner to rub her lower leg lightly up and down in time with her breathing.
- Another wanted her partner to count her breaths out loud and point out to her when she was beyond the number of breaths that meant the halfway point in the contraction.
- Another dealt with her back pain by leaning on the bathroom sink, swaying rhythmically from side to side and moaning, while her partner pressed on her low back.
- Another let her breathing follow the rhythm of her partner's hand moving up and down, "conducting;" she focused entirely on her partner's ring as her guide.
- Another integrated several rituals into one—slow dancing with her partner for every contraction as a helper lightly brushed behind her knees (as a reminder to relax the joint)

at the onset of the contraction; she repeated the words "baby" and "open" out loud; and wanted an ice-cold washcloth to refresh herself between contractions.

Once a woman finds a ritual, she depends on it for many contractions, even hours. Changing the ritual or disturbing it throws her off. Most women change their ritual from time to time in labor, when a change of pace seems necessary. Sudden abandonment of the ritual is a likely sign of progress in the labor.

*Adapted from materials authored by Penny Simkin in the DONA International Birth Doula Training Manual*

# What to Bring to the Hospital or Birth Center

**Small Bag for Labor**
Chap Stick
Massage lotion
Oil for the perineum
Essential oils (Lavender is a good one)
Something to pass the time in early labor (cards, book, etc.)
Fluids for mom (see article "The Birth Marathon: Food & Drink for Labor & Birth")
Snacks for partner
Bathing suit and change of clothes for partner
Toothbrush and toothpaste for partner
Music, Ipod
Birth ball & pump
Plastic container, large enough to hold compresses (e.g., water, washcloth and ice)
T-shirt (or clothing of your choice) to labor in (if desired)
Warm socks
At least two pillows (in colored pillow cases)
10 copies of your Birth Plan

**Suitcase**
Nightgowns (2)
Robe and slippers
Toothbrush and toothpaste
Comb, brush, etc.
Deodorant or other toiletries
Shower cap
Underpants
Nursing bras
Reading/writing materials
Going home clothes (that fit at 6 months)

**For the Baby**
Infant car seat safely installed (have this checked by a certified technician)
Receiving blanket, outdoor blanket
Outfit to wear home, undershirt, booties, cap
Diapers
Diaper wraps or plastic pants (if not using disposables)

# The Birth Marathon—Food & Drink for Labor & Birth

Despite research that concludes that moms should have access to food and drink in labor, many moms birthing in U.S. hospitals today are faced with instructions to not eat solid food and are restricted to ingesting clear liquids only. If labor goes on longer than your blood sugar can hold out and contractions or your energy begin to wane, try the following options. Your overall strategy here is to achieve a stable blood sugar throughout labor. This can be challenging, not just due to restrictive hospital policies and the limitations of what is available on site, but because:

- some women feel nauseous from the onset of labor
- some women respond to pain with nausea and vomiting
- digestion does slow considerably during active labor because blood flow is concentrated to the uterus
- you may not have an appetite
- you may fear vomiting (remember, however, that nausea is one of the symptoms caused by low blood sugar!)

## Strategies

- Some women experience an urge to load up on carbohydrates in the 24-hour period before the onset of active labor, similar to what an athlete may do in preparation for running a marathon on the following day. Go for it! (I had a bread, salad and pasta dinner at a local restaurant 12 hours before my second child was born and never felt nauseated in labor, which started about 5 hours after the meal.) This strategy is especially recommended if you are facing a scheduled induction. You don't want the hard work to hit after you've been essentially fasting for 24 hours or more.

- EAT WHILE YOU ARE STILL AT HOME IN EARLY LABOR. This is key and must be maintained throughout the day. Don't just settle for breakfast and stop there. Eat every 2–3 hours, whatever appeals. You may want to avoid heavy, greasy foods such as pizza or fast foods (which don't digest easily under the best of circumstances).

- Avoid substances that will spike your blood sugar such as pop and other forms of concentrated sugar (read your labels!). These will dehydrate you and ultimately lead to your blood sugar crashing.

- Eat a banana on the way to the birth center/hospital. Despite most TV depictions of how women go into labor (i.e., a sudden contraction alerts her to the need to rush to the hospital where she gives birth soon after on her back, typically involving various emergencies for dramatic effect), most women have plenty of time to take care of themselves at home and head to the birthing center/hospital with little need for high drama.

- During labor, try a variety of the suggestions below, alternating them. A little protein here, some electrolytes there, something sweet to boost your energy, the Pregnancy Tea … you get the idea. That will keep you going if your labor is long. This is especially important for women who might be admitted to the hospital early in labor or whose labor is being induced.

- Drink lots of water, at least 4 ounces per hour throughout your labor, more if it's a hot day and you're sweating a lot. Have your support team help you with this. (Note to partners and doulas: It's your job to encourage the mom to drink throughout her labor. If she is willing to drink, asking for it and consistently taking several gulps when offered, then just keep the supply coming and keep an eye on her to ensure she doesn't stop drinking at some point. However, if the mom is disinterested in drinking and reluctant to do so, then frequent small sips will be necessary. Keep offering!)

- Finally, don't hesitate to accept IV fluids if you can't keep anything down over a long period of time and are getting dehydrated. While most healthy women will not need routine IV fluids, dehydration can cause your labor to be dysfunctional and nonproductive. An IV can turn the picture around and is an appropriate use of medical intervention.

**Raspberry Leaf Tea Labor Cubes**
Before labor begins, make up a VERY strong tea (two quarts of boiling water with 2 cups of dried red raspberry leaves added). Simmer with the lid off for at least 20–30 minutes as the volume reduces considerably. Strain and add ¼ cup of honey (raw is best if possible). Pour into ice cube trays and freeze, adding water if necessary for at least one tray's worth. Store in a zippy bag at home or take with you to the birth center/hospital (usually you can store them in the freezer of the small room refrigerator or in the common "nutrition room" refrigerator). The honey gives mom a boost of energy, while the concentrated raspberry leaves provide minerals and may assist in bringing back strong contractions. In between the contractions, mom can easily crunch the cubes into a satisfying slush.

**Electrolyte-Balanced Sports Drinks**
There are a large variety of sports drinks on the market these days. Avoid the overly-sweet, chemically-generated metallic blue and other colored products not found in nature. See what's available at your local health food store and find something you like. Have 2–3 quarts on hand for labor (your support team will appreciate these as well). I like a product called Recharge and it comes in several flavors.

**Miso Broth**
If you're unfamiliar, miso is a paste made from fermented soybeans. It is high in protein and tastes salty. If you haven't tried miso, there are a number of different flavors available in the refrigerated section of your local health food store. Give them a try and find one you like. The paste can be brought with you to the hospital and kept in the refrigerator. Mix one tablespoon of miso into one cup of hot water. Avoid boiling miso as it kills many of the nutrients. There are

also packets of instant "miso soup" on the market. This is a good option for doulas and midwives to carry with their birth supplies.

## Concentrated Home-Made Chicken or Beef Broth

Place one whole (preferably organic) chicken or a couple of beef bones in a large soup pot. Bring to a boil and spoon off the scum that will rise to the surface over a 10-minute period and discard. Roughly cut up 1 onion, 3 carrots (washed, with skins on) and 3 stalks of celery, including tops. Chop up 2–3 garlic cloves and throw those in too (you can even leave the skins on as a timesaver). Cover and reduce heat, simmering for 1½ hours. Allow cooling and strain out the solids (make chicken salad with the meat). Put in refrigerator overnight so that the layer of fat on top solidifies. In the morning, remove and discard the fat layer, but don't worry if a little is left behind. Return the broth to the stove uncovered and bring to a boil, allowing the liquid to reduce to a rich-colored (and tasty!) broth. Add in salt to taste at the very end. Freeze in small containers to have on hand for labor.

## Herb Tea and Honey

Bring a variety of your favorite herbal teabags and some raw honey with you to the hospital. When energy flags, especially in the second stage of labor, a cup of tea with a generous spoonful of honey can give you the boost you need to get the job done. Ginger tea can settle the stomach if nausea is an issue.

## Hot Drinks

Americans are big on iced drinks, but in many parts of the world, ingesting iced drinks is not recommended. A number of cultures, from China to South America, have prohibitions against iced drinks for women in labor or postpartum. The wise women grandmas-to-be will not allow it. Feed the fire. You are supposed to get hot in labor! You will sweat. You will be uncomfortable. It's okay. It's more efficient.

## Labor Food

Women have been using tubes of concentrated carbohydrates found in the runners' stores (aka "goo"). Lots of flavors, promoted as digesting rapidly and easily while vigorously exercising, and easy to just take a squirt. Be sure and follow up with water as it is very concentrated. Rave reviews from birthing moms.

## Other Labor Foods
- bananas (worth mentioning twice due to portability and high potassium content)
- yogurt or keifer or fruit smoothies
- light foods that appeal

This article was written by Patty Brennan and is excerpted from her cookbook, Whole Family Recipes: For the Childbearing Year & Beyond [www.center4cby.com].

# Cheat Sheet for the Birth Partner

## Early Labor (at home)
- Encourage mom to eat to appetite
- Remind her to drink fluids.
- Help her to REST for the big event (no last-minute housecleaning!).
- Remind mom to keep her bladder empty.
- If labor starts in the middle of the night, encourage mom to go back to sleep.
- Keep mom company and distract her—walk with her, play cards, watch TV, dance, etc.
- Encourage mom to change positions frequently, favoring upright positions.
- Time contractions, from time to time, and keep a written record. (Time from onset of one contraction to the onset of the next one; that is the frequency of the contractions. Also note how long the contraction lasts.) Do this for an hour or so and then put the stopwatch aside. Can check again later if it feels like things are picking up.
- Watch mom for visible signs of tension, especially in response to contractions, and help her to relax (baths, massage, deep breathing, verbal reminders).
- If mom seems anxious, ask her what she needs to feel safe.
- Ask her if there is anything she needs done around the house "to feel ready."
- Keep your care providers and support team updated.
- Realize that if you tell friends and family that you are in labor, you are inviting their energy and possible intrusion into the experience. Would it be better to let them know after the baby is born?
- Protect her from any negative people or influences.
- Tell her how well she is doing.
- Enjoy this time together.

---

*Eat, Drink, Pee, Rest, Sleep, Distraction, Encouragement, Relax, Protect, Emotional Support*

---

## Active Labor
- Eliminate distractions in the environment; add to comfort with pillows, dimmed lights, music, etc.
- Control the presence of visitors, in alignment with your birth plan.
- Help navigate any decisions regarding her care, using your birth plan as a guide.
- Keep lips and mouth moist.
- Give her a back massage.
- Encourage her to drink fluids and urinate at least once per hour.
- Encourage mom to change positions frequently, favoring upright positions.
- Remember the 3 R's—Rhythm, Relaxation, Ritual.
- Recognize when she is coping well (rhythmic movement, relaxation) and protect the ritual.
- Help her find a ritual that works if she is struggling.

- Suggest immersion in water (if she is able) or a shower.
- Tell her you are proud of her.
- Praise her strength.

> *Drink, Pee, Protect, Informed Decision Making, the 3 R's,*
> *Massage, Support, Move, Encourage, Guide, Praise*

## Transition
- Remind her to take one contraction at a time.
- Breathe with her.
- Help her to rest and relax between contractions (big breath out).
- If she panics, move in close, establish eye contact and help her stay focused for every contraction.
- Change the ritual if the one she was using isn't working any more.
- Expect it to get a little hairy; this just means that she is progressing (remind her of this!).
- Remember that this is usually the shortest part of labor.
- Don't give up on her if she gives up on herself.
- Hold intent for her if she has lost it temporarily.
- Validate her feelings.
- Tell her that you love her.

> *Face-to-Face, Breathe, Stay Calm, Hold Intent, Validate, Reassure*

## 2nd Stage/Pushing
- Help her find the most comfortable and productive position
- Whisper words of encouragement. "You're doing just fine." "Just like that."
- Encourage her to rest between contractions.
- Remind care providers about any key items in the birth plan related to 2nd stage and immediate postpartum care for the baby (e.g., hot compresses to perineum, skin-to-skin, delayed cord clamping, etc.).
- Enjoy your baby!

> *Positioning Support, Encouragement, Advocacy, Delight*

## 3rd Stage/Delivery of Placenta
- Stay focused on the mom and the birth (it's not over yet; phone calls can wait).

- If she is reluctant, remind her that there are no bones in the placenta ("Almost done.").
- Give her a drink of something sweet.
- If she is shaky, ask the nurse to get her warm blankets.
- Encourage skin-to-skin contact with the baby.
- Continue to advocate for birth plan, as needed.
- Enjoy your baby!

*Focus, Drinks, Warmth, Protect, Celebrate*

## Immediate Postpartum Recovery (First Two Hours)

- Keep mom and baby together, skin-to-skin.
- Baby will likely want to latch at the breast if given access. Ask for privacy if you like.
- Now you can make your calls! (Make an assessment whether or not you want visitors right away.)
- Take pictures.
- Have a meal.
- Celebrate!
- REST.

*Skin-to-Skin, Breastfeeding, Privacy, Eat, Pictures, Celebrate, Rest*

## If Things Don't Go as Planned

- Help with informed decision making. Remember the questions:
    1. How will this help mom or baby?
    2. Can you describe the procedure involved?
    3. What are the risks or unintended consequences?
    4. Urgency? What are the consequences of giving it more time?
    5. Choices? Is there anything else that can be tried instead?
- Continue to advocate for pieces of the Birth Plan that can still be accomplished (e.g., skin-to-skin immediately after a cesarean delivery may be possible, even while mom is still on the operating table).
- Try to minimize the down side of any medical interventions (e.g., she does not need to lie flat on her back in bed just because she has fetal monitors strapped on or even an epidural in place).
- Understand that you are doing your best and that birth is unpredictable. Hang in there.

*Informed Consent, Advocacy, Adaptation, Stay with It*

## Additional Suggestions for Partners

- Wear comfortable clothing and shoes. You could be on your feet for a long time.
- Bring a bathing suit or pair of shorts that you can wear in the shower (or birth tub, if that is part of your plan).
- Bring a change of clothes.
- Pack food and drink for yourself.
- Keep your breath fresh by bringing a toothbrush and toothpaste.
- Bring your birth plan and have a good understanding of mom's wishes and desires for the birth.
- Recruit additional help for the labor room if you are feeling like you could use some support. A mother, sister, aunt, close friend or doula could be that person for you.

BRING: *Comfortable Clothing, Food & Drink, Breath Freshener, Birth Plan, More Help(?)*

# Emotional Birthing ~ Partner Exercise

## Instructions

1. Read two stories, *Safer Birth in a Barn?* and *Story of Mama Elephant*.

2. Next, each partner works through the questions in the Partner Exercises.

3. The Affirmations and Visualizations sheets are included immediately following the exercise sheets, for your reference.

4. Finally, share your responses and thoughts with your partner.

## Safer Birth in a Barn?
*By Beth Barbeau* [www.VisitIndigo.com]

Our deeper understandings of birth can come to us from the most unexpected sources and at the most unanticipated times. One of my most visceral "light-bulb" experiences came in New Mexico in the early 1990s when I was taking a break from midwifery and selling health insurance to self-employed individuals.

One day, I drove several hours to meet with the general manager of an immense horse farm, hoping to sell a large policy to cover his many farm hands. I ended up wandering through some of the buildings, searching for my appointment. I mentally noted as I passed that one of the stalls exuded energy that felt like birth. Peeking in, I found a swollen mare pacing restlessly in the afternoon quiet, deeply breathing and blowing.

We were in the middle of the insurance presentation about an hour later when an assistant breathlessly burst in saying that "so and so" was foaling! The manager stood up immediately and said, "Do you want to see a foal born?" He was startled when I asked if it was the mare I had glimpsed earlier. When I shared that I had trained as a midwife and it just "felt and smelled of birth," he brightened and lost his taciturn ways, suddenly eager to talk about what he loved.

Until the next few minutes, I did not fully understand that I was in a very unusual place—a stud farm for some of the most valuable horses in the world. This particular unborn foal was worth about three million dollars and was expected to be of much greater value after birth because it shared lineage with two Triple Crown winners. The horseman explained what I was about to see as we hurried over. He was adamant about his instructions, stressing the careful attention to detail needed to protect the well-being of this babe of breath-taking value.

*"Don't let the mare see you; crouch here in the hallway where you can peek over the half wall of the foaling box—the stress of seeing strangers at this time could put the foal in danger!"*

*"The only person allowed near the mare is her familiar stable lad; even her vet is crouched as small as possible in the corner." (And he was, hunched on his heels, silent and still, head and eyes downcast.)*

*"We keep the lights dimmed because bright lights agitate and distract the laboring mare."*

*"You'll see that we've removed her halter and lead—you would never restrict the movement of a birthing mare; foals have been lost for less! She must be free to move any way she wants."*

*"She's been in this box stall (when not out to pasture) for weeks, because she must be in a familiar environment to birth smoothly."*

*"There is her usual water and hay in the stall—never strict their food in labor!"*

*"Don't say a word. Any sound might disrupt the birth and a disruption puts the foal in danger."*

With these admonishments ringing in my ears, I crouched in the dim, silent passageway outside the birthing box with several others. We watched the mare birth a huge colt with grace, barely pausing in her pacing as he slid with a thump to the floor. All was quiet and still in the long minutes afterwards as the colt organized his breathing, gathered himself and finally staggered up. He was so unusually large and long-legged that he stood on his ankles; his cartilage was too soft to support his weight. Still, the horseman was elated with the outcome, passing off the odd and worrisome appearance with a "give him time, he'll work it out."

## Story of Mama Elephant

When an elephant went into labor in an American zoo, the zookeepers put her in her own enclosure, isolating her from the other elephants. As her labor progressed, however, the elephant became distressed and began thrashing about violently. Recognizing that something was going terribly wrong, the officials quickly telephoned a European zoo where an elephant had recently given birth successfully. When the Americans described what was happening, the Europeans were shocked. "Where are her midwives?" they demanded. "Where are the other female elephants to help with the delivery?"

The Americans immediately complied with the European's instructions. As soon as they were allowed into the area with the birthing mother, the other female elephants rushed to her and began to assist her, stroking her with their trunks, calming her with their presence and helping her to complete her labor. After the newborn elephant emerged, the midwives cleaned the baby and took care of her while the mother rested.

The art of women supporting women in childbirth is seen not only throughout the history of humankind, but in the animal world as well. Elephants in the wild have midwives who surround them in a circle during their labor. The elephant midwives may care for the pregnant elephants throughout their long gestation of 21–22 months, in labor and through infancy.

An elephant's labor ranges in length from 5 minutes to 60 hours. The average length of labor is 11 hours.

## Emotional Birthing/Mom—Partner Exercise

### Birth as a Rite of Passage

A rite of passage typically involves a ceremony that marks important transitional periods in a person's life such as birth, puberty, marriage, having children and death. Considering the gravity of bringing a child from your body and into this world, what could be some fun or special ways of celebrating or honoring birth as a rite of passage on the day of the birth while you are in labor?

### Emotional Coping

Throughout our childbirth preparation programs, we discuss variations in the physical and emotional process of birth, present a variety of coping techniques and give partners tools to help support you. Putting all of that aside, what do you think you can do for yourself on the day of the birth that will help you cope? What tools do you have to jump through any emotional hurdles you may encounter?

### Affirmations

Refer to the Affirmations handout. Highlight and discuss the phrases that resonate with you. Why are these important to be reminded of (by partner) and repeat/think to yourself while you are in labor? Any others that you would like to hear that are not on the list?

### Visualizations

Read through the visualizations and choose some that you think might work for you. Discuss with your partner what you think might work for you and why.

### Sensuality in Birth

Remember that birth is an extension of the sensual energy that created your baby in the first place. Natural childbirth is the grand climax. This is when the energy peaks and flows powerfully through you, bringing your baby into life. As your birthing time begins, the flood gate swings open and this powerful flame, which has so patiently waited inside, is set free. How you choose to interpret and use this amazingly powerful energy is up to you, and can be the difference between whether your natural childbirth is experienced as pain or pleasure. "You are responsible for your own orgasm"— meaning you are responsible for your own experience. Most women will agree that you can have horrible sex or amazing sex just based on how you choose to interpret and respond to it. It's all about how much you can allow yourself to release into it. How open are you to the sensuality of your being for this birth? Think about places and situations in both your home and/or hospital where you would feel comfortable letting your sensuality flow. And what could your partner do to protect your space and/or help you feel comfortable letting go completely?

## Emotional Birthing/Dads or Partner—Partner Exercise

### Privacy and Environment

After reading the story of the elephant mother and the one about the birthing horse, what thoughts come to mind about the level of privacy your partner might need for birthing?

It has been said that "holding the space" for the laboring woman is the most important gift a partner can give on the day of the birth. What does this statement mean to you? How can you "hold the space" for your partner?

Think about some specific things you can control in her environment (home, birth center, or hospital) that might make it an inviting place to labor and birth.

### Encouragement and Praise

After reading about Encouragement in Labor, what are your thoughts on what might work for your partner? How is she a birthing warrior (strong and capable) in your mind? How can you remind her of this strength and wisdom she has inside?

### Freaking Out/Panic

What if your wife/partner begins to panic? She might say things such as "I can't do this." How can you help her reset her emotional state so she can accept the intensity of this birth? (Hint: think about your demeanor, her breathing, her environment.)

**Caring for Yourself**

There is so much focus on supporting your partner through this process. How can you make sure your needs are met during the birthing process, especially if it is long?

**Sensuality in Birth**

*"The physical expression of love can be an enormous help. Kissing, cuddling, sensual caress, massage and nipple stimulation can all have a positive effect on the progression of birth. When you and your partner are able to remain conscious of allowing your love to flow freely without being restricted, then birth is more likely to flow freely without being restricted."*

What do you think about this statement? Have you ever viewed birth as sensual? What kinds of sensual support might you offer your lover as she cycles through her birthing experience?

# The Value of Affirmations

Our values and beliefs influence what happens to us by aligning our energy with them and making it more likely that they will manifest in our lives. Much of our life has a self-fulfilling character. We seem to attract what we fear, or we can often say, "I knew that would happen to me." Since what we say about ourselves (positive or negative) strongly influences what actually unfolds in our lives, it is possible to take advantage of this by creating or using positive affirmations. Repeating or writing affirmations such as the following can help you to realize their truth and to identify and release any blocks from the past that may stand in the way of these statements manifesting in your life. By employing affirmations, we can reprogram deep-seated, often subconscious, patterns in our lives that are not serving us well.

## Some Pregnancy Affirmations
- My body is beautiful and strong.
- My baby is growing beautiful and strong.
- I am and will be a good parent to my child(ren).
- The Universe loves and supports me and my baby.
- My baby and I are ready for the Divine Plan of our lives to unfold.
- The baby is naturally developing and doing just what he/she should.
- Pregnancy is natural, normal, healthy, and safe for me and my baby.
- My baby knows when it is time to be born.
- My body will go into labor on its own, at the perfect time.
- I am doing a great job taking care of myself and the baby.

## Some Birth Affirmations
- My body knows how to give birth and I will let it.
- Contractions help my baby to be born.
- Each contraction brings me closer to meeting my baby.
- Strong contractions are good ones.
- I am strong and I can let my contractions be strong.
- I am calm and relaxed. My baby feels my calmness and shares it.
- The baby and I are rested and ready for the work we will do.
- With each contraction my cervix is dilating a little more.
- My contractions are massaging the baby and hugging him/her.
- The baby is descending naturally.
- The baby's head fits perfectly in my pelvis.
- I am opening.
- My tissues are stretching beautifully, just as they should.
- I accept the healthy pain of labor, if and when it is here.
- I feel the love of those who are helping me.
- I attract wonderful people to support me in labor.

- My health care providers are very respectful of my wishes.
- I send love to my baby and call him/her to my arms.

**Some Postpartum Affirmations**
- My body is beautiful and strong.
- I am proud of all that I have accomplished.
- My body knows how to make milk.
- My body is making the perfect amount of breast milk.
- I know how to nurse my baby.
- I am adjusting to life with my new baby.
- I share in the strength and wisdom of all mothers.

**Suggestions for Working with Affirmations**

- Work with one or more every day. The best times are just before sleeping, before starting the day or when you are feeling troubled.

- Write each affirmation 10 or 20 times on a sheet of paper, leaving space in the right-hand margin of the page for the "emotional response." As you write the affirmation down on the left side of the page, jot down whatever thoughts, considerations, beliefs, fears or emotions come to your mind. Keep repeating the affirmation and notice how the responses on the right side change.

- Put specific names and situations into the affirmation. Include your name in the affirmation. Say and write each affirmation in the first, second and third person. "I (your name) love myself. You (your name) love yourself. (Your name) now loves herself."

- Play with the vocabulary in the affirmation. Make it personal and meaningful. Be specific about your desired result.

- Record your affirmations and play them back when you can. A good time is while driving or when going to bed.

- Try looking in the mirror and saying the affirmations to yourself out loud. Keep saying them until you are able to see yourself with a relaxed, happy expression. Keep saying them until you eliminate all facial tension and grimaces.

- Sit across from a partner, each of you in a straight chair with your hands on your thighs and knees barely touching. Say the affirmation to your partner until you are comfortable doing it. Your partner can observe your body language carefully. If you squirm, fidget or are unclear, you do not pass. He or she should not allow you to go on until you say the affirmation very clearly, without contrary body reactions and upsets. Then your partner says them back to you, using the second person and your name. Continue until you can receive them without embarrassment. This is harder than it sounds!

- Don't give up! If you ever get to a point where you begin to feel upset, shaky or afraid about something negative you discover, don't panic. Keep on writing the applicable affirmation over and over until your mind takes on a new thought. As it does, the negativity will fade away and you will feel lighter and better. Remember, it is just as easy to think positively as negatively. In fact, it is easier. Negative thinking actually takes more effort.

- Don't be afraid to experiment. Affirmations can be useful in all areas of your life—for problems at work, problems with health, personal growth ...

# Visualizations for Birth

Visualization is a great relaxation technique for nearly everyone. It can be done in many situations and has great potential to be very individualized. When we talk about visualization, most people think of things like reading scenarios of walking through the forest or lying on the beach listening to waves. That can be a visualization exercise. However, what works best is usually something personal.

Many people enjoy reliving a positive experience, a date, a vacation, their wedding. This is done by the retelling of the story by your partner. Be sure to include all of the details to actually help you remember—sights, smells, tastes and sounds. Using all of the senses is important.

Explaining what is going on in the body and using those images as a relaxation tool is also beneficial. For example, remind the mother that what she is feeling is her cervix opening and provide a visual image, such as a flower bud opening. Some women will even choose a single, inanimate object. It might be a photo, a special relaxation card or whatever works.

Visualization for relaxation is a basic skill for labor and childbirth. Many childbirth classes teach visualization as a way to promote relaxation and reduce pain and fear in labor. Following the fear-tension-pain cycle, we know that to help reduce pain, we need to reduce fear and tension.

Here is a simple exercise for visualization:

- Begin by taking a few, deep abdominal breaths. This will help you release tension and center yourself. Then picture an image that represents tension, this could be any image, but the exercise will be most effective if you choose a picture that represents something to you from your own life. Examples might be a closed cervix or fist, a contraction or a crying baby.

- Continue the deep breathing as you find this tension image. As soon as you have focused on an image, begin to find a way to relax the image. That is, have the cervix soften and open in your mind; watch the contraction work and then ease; or have the crying baby brought skin to skin and calm.

- You can use this during contractions or afterward as you try to scan your body for tension after the contraction is over. When you are done with this visualization exercise, consider repeating an affirmation to praise yourself and reinforce the relaxing thoughts.

# Encouragement in Labor

During labor, one of the most power tools of the coach is the ability to ensure the mother that she is doing well and to encourage her to continue what she is already doing. You may not believe it, but many a laboring mother has been helped by three little words, "You're doing great!" It sounds too simple to be true, but it is.

During active labor, the mother may not realize how far she has come. She is literally taking her labor one contraction at a time and, unlike those supporting her, she may not see it as one contraction closer to the birth. She may not even recognize that she has a significant portion of her labor behind her. That is one of the reasons a coach is so important. The coach becomes the mother's "eyes and ears," watching what is happening and letting the mother know where she is. Comments such as "I can't do this!" can be calmed by responses such as, "but you've been doing this for an hour and you're doing great." Suddenly, the mother will have a new-found confidence to continue.

Transition is a time of confusion for a mother. She cannot get comfortable and she doesn't seem to know what to do. Coping techniques that were working may suddenly stop helping. She may not even remember that she is in labor for a baby. It is at this point that the reassuring words of her coach can help a woman most. She will need to be reminded how close she is to pushing and to holding her baby. She will also need to be reminded what to do. She may not remember for more than a few seconds, so repeat yourself without getting frustrated. Looks of panic on the mother can be responded to with, "I'm right here, we're almost done."

What are the magic words of encouragement that will help the mother? That will depend on who she is and what your relationship is to her. In some instances, "I love you" will be reassuring. In other cases, "You're doing perfect, it's beautiful to watch you" will reassure her. As coach, you should know the mother well enough to know what will relax and reassure her. You may also try repeating an encouraging phrase several times. Lines such as the following, said to the mother during a contraction, can give her something to focus on, while reassuring her that what is happening is normal.

I love you.
You're doing so well.
That's it … That's the way.
You're doing it!
You are so strong—strong enough for this.
You're working with the contractions so well.
You are relaxing beautifully.
It's okay to cry.
That was a good one!
I'm right here.
I will help you.

You can do it.

Say with me, "I can do it."

Each contraction is bringing our baby closer.

We will meet our baby soon!

I'm proud of you.

Let's just get through this one.

Perfect, just perfect.

The baby is moving down, the baby will be here soon.

You're doing exactly what you need to be doing.

The baby is trying to come out. You are helping her come out.

The stronger it feels, the better it works.

You are doing so well.

Your body is working perfectly. Everything is working perfectly.

# Fears in a Box ~ Partner Exercise

You and your partner each write down your top three fears about the upcoming birth and becoming a parent (or adding another child to your existing family).

Hand your fears sheet to your partner. Explore each fear. Be curious.

What is behind the fear? Is this fear stemming from a belief that you have? What is that belief? Where did it come from (you probably have good reasons for it)? Is there a way you can reframe that belief?

Is there a way to address this fear proactively? What steps can you take?

Can you create a vision for your birth or for after the baby is born, that reframes or transforms this fear in a positive way? (See also, *The Value of Affirmations* on p. 84).

Brainstorm ways your partner can help you with your fear(s). What makes it less scary for you? What would make it worse?

When we take our fears out of the box, we rob them of some of their power, because they are brought up to the conscious level. Then we can address them and others can provide support as we move through them.

# Bishop's Score for Induction of Labor

This is the table used to determine how successful an induction of labor might be. It is recommended that the Bishop's Score be greater than 9 for induction to be successful. To ensure your own induction's success rate, inquire about your Bishop's Score. The unfortunate reality is that there are inductions being performed with scores as low as 2 that make induction very difficult and success rates low. Induction with a low Bishop's Score decreases a woman's ability to cope with the increased pain of induction and increased length of labor. When combined with artificial rupture of membranes (in an effort to boost the success rate), the risk of infection for mom and baby, as well as the incidence of cesarean delivery, go up. We encourage you to make informed decisions for both you and your baby!

**Bishop's Score**
0, 1, 2, or 3 points are assigned for each parameter listed.

**Position of Cervix**
0    Posterior (towards the back)
1    Mid-position
2    Anterior (towards the front)

**Consistency of Cervix**
0    Firm
1    Medium
2    Soft (ripe)

**Effacement of Cervix**
0    0-30%
1    40-50%
2    60-70%
3    >80%

**Dilation of Cervix**
0    Closed/0 cm
1    1-2 cm
2    3-4 cm
3    >5 cm

**Baby's Station (degree of engagement in mom's pelvis)**
0    -3
1    -2
2    -1, 0
3    +1, +2

## Cervical Sensations
0      None
1      Slight
2      Strong and frequent
3      Coordinated with some or all toning contractions

## + Vaginal Secretions
0      No increase
1      Increased mucus
2      Increased with bloody mucus

## + Toning Contractions
0      None to slight
1      Mild
2      Strong, sporadic, frequent
3      Almost regular, visible on abdominal observation

## Modifiers: Add 1 point to score for each of the following
- Preeclampsia
- Each prior vaginal delivery

## Subtract 1 point from score for each of the following:
- Postdates pregnancy
- Nulliparity (never having borne children)
- Premature or prolonged rupture of membranes

## Total Score = sum of all points for each parameter

## Interpreting Your Score
7 or less: Do **not** attempt induction without ripening the cervix first
9 or more: Favorable to attempt induction
12 or more: You are quite ready for labor or in early labor; consider if there is anything you need to feel ready

## Note
+ All items with a "plus sign" are added by Anne Frye, *Holistic Midwifery Volume II,* and have been proven helpful from a midwifery-model perspective. All others are original components of the Bishop's Score. If only using only the original components, then 7 and above is considered a favorable score.

# Active Management of Third Stage of Labor

## Definitions and Related Facts

### Postpartum hemorrhage and complications of third stage of labor
- Blood loss in excess of 500 ml, with severe postpartum hemorrhage being loss of 1,000 ml or more, and very severe being a loss of 2,500 ml or more.
- Anemia in the mother can pre-exist or be the result of hemorrhage; severe cases may necessitate a blood transfusion.
- Postpartum hemorrhage is the main cause of maternal death in a number of countries, the vast majority of which occur in the developing world.

### Active management of third stage
- 10 units IM Pitocin administered to all mothers within one minute of delivery.
- Early clamping and cutting of the umbilical cord, often before the cord ceases to pulse (thereby cutting off the transfer to the baby of his/her full blood volume).
- Wait one minute, after clamping the cord, and initiate controlled cord traction for delivery of the placenta.

### Expectant management of third stage
- Signs of placental separation are awaited and the placenta is delivered spontaneously via normal uterine contractions.
- May involve nipple stimulation by putting the baby to breast immediately after delivery, stimulating an oxytocin surge in the mother.
- Medical interventions that interfere with the body's natural oxytocin release may reduce the effectiveness of the physiological process (i.e., oxytocin release can be inhibited by anxiety and excess adrenaline, oxytocin augmentation in labor, and administration of epidural or narcotic analgesia).
- The umbilical cord is left intact until it has ceased pulsing and baby has received his/her full blood volume.
- Uterotonic drugs are used only in cases of excess bleeding.

## What does the evidence say?
Medical recommendations in favor of active management over expectant management of third stage of labor are based on an updated Cochrane Review of seven studies involving 8,247 women. For all women, irrespective of their risk of severe bleeding, active management protocols reduced the incidence of severe postpartum blood loss, maternal blood transfusions and postpartum anemia. At the same time, the following statistically significant negative effects of active management were noted:

- Increase in mother's blood pressure, afterpains, vomiting and use of drugs for pain relief; these effects are apparently due to administration of a specific uterotonic (choice of drug used, specifically ergometrine).
- Increase in the number of women returning to the hospital ER after discharge (between 24 hours and up to 6 weeks) due to bleeding (3.8% of patients requiring additional treatment in the active management group vs. 3.1% in the expectant management group).
- Decrease in newborn birth weight due to early cord clamping leading to a 20% reduction in the baby's overall blood volume. *(The World Health Organization now recommends active management with delayed cord clamping—allowing baby's blood that is in the placenta to return to the baby's circulation—to reduce the likelihood of anemia in the newborn. However, in many healthcare settings, this recommendation is not followed.)*

## Discussion by Authors

"The previous authors of this review [2011] recommended active management of the third stage due to the benefit identified in terms of reduced incidence of severe bleeding. We agree that bleeding is a very important component when balancing the benefits and harms of active compared to expectant management of the third stage of labour. However, we consider that the number of harms caused by active management also deserve consideration. In particular, the increased rate of hypertension, increased numbers of mothers returning to hospital due to bleeding and the possible decrease in average blood volume of newborns reflected in the lower birthweight for babies where the mother has received active management of the third stage, are of concern. *In the population of women at low risk of bleeding such harms are of more concern as there was no statistical evidence that severe bleeding was reduced by active management.*" [Emphasis added.]

## Authors' Conclusions

"Healthcare providers should, therefore, present information to all women in the antenatal period on the advantages and disadvantages of both methods of third-stage management to facilitate their discussion and informed choice of care. This information should include not only the benefits of active management … but also the harms to the mother … In addition, information regarding the effects on the baby of early versus deferred cord clamping should be provided…."

## Source
Cochrane Review, *Active versus expectant management for women in the third stage of labor.* Cochrane Library 2015 Issue 3.

# Commentary by Patty Brennan

**Question for Parents to Consider.** For low-risk women, especially those experiencing drug free labors, do the benefits of active management of third stage of labor outweigh the risks? *Parents are encouraged to discuss the benefits and risks of active management with their midwife or doctor as it applies uniquely to their situation.*

**Things Are Happening Fast & Informed Consent.** In my experience, in healthcare settings where active management is routine, informed consent for this practice is rare. Two specific pieces of active management—early cord clamping and administration of an uterotonic drug—are usually completed within a minute after birth. Therefore many parents (being somewhat distracted) may not even notice what is being done until after the fact. Parents who prefer an expectant management approach will need to discuss their preferences with their care provider, express their wishes in a birth plan and then be prepared to advocate for their preferences at the birth. Keep in mind that whomever you discussed this with prenatally is not necessarily the same person who will be attending your birth.

**Mixed Management Option.** Further study is needed on the possibility of a "mixed management option" but should be considered based on the mother's risk factors. A mixed management system might be most beneficial for someone with a high risk birth. For example, for someone with low iron, one option might look like this: "IM Pitocin immediately following the birth to decrease the chance of hemorrhage (active management), delayed cord clamping to allow the baby to receive his/her full blood volume from the placenta (expectant management), and careful cord traction once the cord is done pulsing to ensure there isn't excessive bleeding behind the placenta (mild active management)."

**Delayed Cord Clamping.** In a post on Lamaze International's *Science and Sensibility* blog, pediatrician Dr. Mark Sloan examines common objections to delayed cord clamping and what the evidence says about its benefits. Dr. Sloan concludes, *"The evidence of benefit from delayed cord clamping is so compelling that the burden of proof must now lie with those who wish to continue the practice of immediate clamping, rather than with those who prefer—as nature intended—to wait."*

**Prevent Anemia.** If active management of third stage is being promoted as a benefit to anemic mothers (those with low blood levels of iron who might suffer more from even a normal blood loss at their birth), then let's become as proactive as possible about preventing and treating anemia prior to the birth through proper nutrition and supplementation (see p. 20 for more information).

**The Midwifery Model of Care.** Finally, in my opinion, active management of third stage of labor is inconsistent with the Midwifery Model of Care [www.cfmidwifery.org]. Specifically, it violates the basic tenet of respect for the birth process as it unfolds uniquely, as well as the belief that birth is a normal life process for which women's bodies are well designed. This is to be distinguished from the medical model approach wherein birth is viewed as an emergency waiting to happen and interference with the normal process is common.

# Steps for Reducing the Need for a Cesarean

- Eat properly, get plenty of rest and exercise, and avoid undue stress.

- Develop trust in the birth process; take personal responsibility for the birth rather than expecting the doctor/midwife to take care of everything.

- Avoid all routine or "just-in-case" interventions; if a clear problem exists, use the least invasive interventions first.

- Choose supportive providers and birth environments, even if it means changing late in pregnancy.

- Use alternative treatments for the four major indications for cesarean, together responsible for about 80% of all cesareans. These are previous cesarean, prolonged labor, fetal distress and breech presentation.

## Alternative Treatments for Prolonged Labor

- Patience and emotional support; slow progress is not inherently dangerous; arbitrary time limits are inappropriate; the diagnosis should not be made before active labor (cervix 4–6 cm and effaced, contractions regular, painful and progressive)

- Ambulation and position changes

- Help with relaxation, including massage, warm water, mental imagery, slow deep breathing and other means

- Nipple stimulation to increase natural oxytocin

- Avoid epidural anesthesia or medication, or let it wear off when second stage is reached or if progress stops.

- Meet fluid and calorie needs; total fasting in labor stresses both mother and baby

- Physiological pushing, in an upright position, only with the mother's reflexive urges, with an open mouth and throat

## To Minimize Fetal Distress, AVOID:

- Supine or back reclining positions (less than 45 degrees from the horizontal)
- Artificial rupture of membranes, except for specific medical need
- Sedation and anesthesia
- Pushing with prolonged breath holding
- Continuous electronic fetal monitoring in low-risk labor; fetal scalp sampling is advised to confirm distress

## Alternatives for Breech Presentation

- Attempt to turn the baby before labor through postural exercises, external cephalic version, or acupuncture.
- Vaginal breech birth by skilled attendant for full-term, normal-sized frank and complete breech babies, without hyper-extended head.
- See www.SpinningBabies.com for more alternative approaches.

## Other Steps to Reduce Risk of Cesarean

- Be a good consumer; shop around for your midwife or doctor. Ask what the cesarean rate is for your caregiver and for your place of birth.
- Take personal responsibility for yourself and your pregnancy through excellent nutrition, prenatal care, self-education and decision making.
- Avoid induction of labor.
- Write a Birth Plan; make sure it is in your chart at the hospital.
- Stay home until active labor is established.
- Don't go alone! Take your well-prepared partner and a professional doula; it's your best investment in cesarean prevention.
- Get up to urinate at least once per hour.
- Change positions frequently—active birth!
- Walk, walk and walk some more.
- Eat and drink to appetite and thirst.
- Avoid all drugs—anesthesia and/or analgesia.
- Avoid IVs and minimize use of electronic fetal monitor.
- If you want a VBAC (vaginal birth after cesarean), find a practitioner who has a high success rate.

# All about Birth Plans

## What is a Birth Plan?

The short answer is that the birth plan is a *tool to facilitate communication.* It is a written description of how you would like to be supported during labor, delivery, and immediately postpartum. It also includes your preferences for the baby during these times. Ideally, a birth plan facilitates communication on a number of levels:

- Between the mother and her partner
- Between the couple and their doula and/or other members of the support team
- Between the couple and their medical care providers

A birth plan is only useful or helpful to the extent that it *actually* facilitates good communication, helping everyone to be on the same page.

> ### What a Birth Plan is Not
> ✓ A script for how your labor and birth will unfold
> ✓ A contract between you and your health care providers
> ✓ A list of procedures you want to avoid
> ✓ More than two pages of information

Planning for labor may seem overwhelming when you consider all the options that are available to you. You may wonder about the value of it, since you can't really plan how your labor will unfold and it's not realistic to plan for every possible contingency (your birth plan would be ten pages along and no one would actually read it!). Your birth plan is an introduction to you and how your support team (medical and otherwise) can best support you and your baby through this experience. It might explain what pain relief techniques you would like to try, what interventions you would like to avoid or what atmosphere you would like to cultivate in the labor room. It can help to set the tone for your birth.

Many women today are attended by doctors and midwives who work in large group practices. You may have an excellent relationship with one particular doctor or midwife, but there is no guarantee that she/he will be the same person who attends you in labor. And no matter how good your prenatal communication and relationship is with your doctor or midwife, you do not know the nurses at the hospital and they do not know you. A birth plan helps people get to know you at a time when you may not be in a frame of mind to introduce yourself and explain all of your needs and preferences.

During labor, if situations arise in which a decision must be made, it is easy for a nurse, doula or coach to check your birth plan for guidance. It lets them know what options you would like to try and what options you would like to avoid if possible.

## How to Write a Birth Plan

### Understand your options.
The first step in writing a birth plan is to find out what your options are. Different doctors will give you different choices for handling the same situation. Different hospitals or birth centers will vary in environment, protocols and available options. Review the **Birth Plan Checklist** included here. Read through the list and determine what options appeal to you and what options you don't think you want. You can use this list to find out what your caregiver feels comfortable with. You should also take the Birth Plan Checklist on a hospital/birth center tour to find out how the policies may affect your options. Ask lots of questions on your tour, even if you are the only one asking questions! Some hospital tour guides may adopt an approach that is best summarized as "how to be a good patient in our hospital." When they understand that you are interested in all of your options, they should be able to switch gears and accommodate you. If you are not satisfied with the options available with your current caregiver/place of birth, then you may want to explore other choices available in your area.

### Examine your feelings and consider your priorities.
Once you know what choices are available to you, it is important to determine how you feel about the options. Some things will be very important and others will seem small or unimportant. There is no right or wrong; it is simply a matter of understanding who you are and how you want things handled. You may find that there are several options that you feel very strongly about. In this case, it might be helpful to use the **Ideal Birth Worksheet** (below) to work through your feelings and rank your choices according to level of importance to you. Both the mother and her partner (if any) need to decide what things are important to them and then discuss their feelings and make any necessary compromises. In the written birth plan, list your choices in order of priority, most important first.

### Determine whether you can get what you want.
As you create your birth plan, be sure and bring it with you to prenatal visits with your doctor or midwife. It is important to begin this process of claiming ownership of your birth during the prenatal period and to begin a discussion with your chosen care provider. The provider can let you know if your requests are realistic, likely to be honored, or even possible within the context of your chosen birth place and given your personal circumstances and medical history. In some cases, you may learn that your care provider does not particularly want to enter into a discussion about your preferences, seems impatient with the entire subject, or flatly states that they cannot support your choices. This will help you determine if your chosen caregiver is the best match for you. If you are not getting a receptive response, consider whether there is room for negotiation and compromise. You are the customer and you are paying the bill. You have some power here, but you will only be as powerful as you believe yourself to be.

**Prepare for a positive experience.**

Be sure to phrase your final birth plan in a pleasant and polite tone. Do not present your preferences as a list of demands. This can help everyone feel more confident and increase your chances of having the birth experience you want.

---

### Birth Plan Tips

✓ Make it short and easy to read.
✓ Divide it in two sections—one for labor and birth and one for postpartum mother-baby care.
✓ Put the most important items first.
✓ Use positive, flexible language (e.g., how you would like to be supported rather than what you don't want people to do).
✓ If you use a template, inject some personality into it.

---

## Choices Regarding Immediate Postpartum Care of the Newborn

Expectant parents are encouraged to consider their preferences regarding the following medical procedures and protocols commonly used with the newborn and to begin a dialogue with their care provider prior to the birth. As you sort out your priorities, you can begin to incorporate your preferences into a Birth Plan. For a hospital birth, typically it is the labor and delivery nurse's job to see that routine procedures are accomplished. If it is important to you to do some things differently than her protocols may require, then it is essential that you get her on board with your plan.

**Do you have preferences about any of the following?**
- Delay cord clamping until the cord has stopped pulsating.
- Refrain from routine suctioning of the baby and provide only if/when necessary.
- Allow for immediate, undisturbed, skin-to-skin contact between mom and baby.
- Stabilize baby's temperature with skin-to-skin on mom or dad rather than using warming table.
- Delay all routines until one hour postpartum (e.g., weighing, measuring, eye drops, etc.).
- Perform routine procedures bedside or even while mom is holding baby, if possible.
- Allow mom and baby time to figure out breastfeeding on their own. Provide support only if asked to do so. Care providers should ask for permission before doing any hands-on breastfeeding support techniques.
- Allow parents to be involved with giving baby his/her first bath; or have it done bedside; or delay until parents are ready.
- Rub vernix "in" rather than "off."

**These procedures are routines, but may be negotiable:**
- Administration of Vitamin K within first hour after birth; may need to request a waiver form
- Blood sugar checks (heel poke), especially indicated for 9+ pound babies; may request to keep baby at breast as an alternative (if baby is not breastfeeding, supplementation may be required to prevent dangerous drop in baby's blood sugar)

**These procedures are required by state law:**
- Antibiotic drops in eyes within first hour after birth (prevention against possible gonorrhea infection that can result in blindness in the newborn); parents may be able to sign a waiver in some care settings.
- Newborn Screening (heel poke for blood samples); very difficult to opt out of this one; see Limitations to Parental Rights below.

**These procedures require explicit parental consent (meaning you have the right to postpone or decline and they will not be done without your expressed consent):**

- Circumcision
- Hepatitis B vaccine; can be delayed until 6 weeks and still be in compliance with American Academy of Pediatricians (AAP) recommendations.

**Limitations to Parental Rights**

In the United States, parents do not retain the legal right to decline recommended medical treatments for their minor children. So, once a family interfaces with the medical care system, they are at risk of losing ultimate decision-making power over their child's medical care. Of course, many doctors will include parents in treatment choices and decisions. However, if parents are refusing what doctors believe to be lifesaving treatment (e.g., antibiotics or blood transfusions), doctors are able to get a court order granting them legal custody of the child on the basis of "medical neglect" on the part of the parents. These situations can become quite contentious, but the courts typically come down on the side of the medical professionals rather than the parents.

**Get a Second Opinion**

If treatments are being recommended for your newborn, especially treatments that require re-hospitalization of the baby or a disruption in breastfeeding (e.g., for jaundice), consider bringing in your private pediatrician for a second opinion. After all, this is the person who is going to be following your baby's care and it makes sense to involve them sooner, rather than later, if an issue is being raised by the hospital's neonatal staff.

**Consider Early Discharge**

If your birth went well, meaning mom feels pretty good and the baby is healthy, then you may want to consider leaving the hospital environment sooner rather than later. This will work especially well if you have a knowledgeable helper at home—perhaps your mom, a doula or an experienced friend. It is a myth that anyone "gets more rest" in the hospital and no one would ever argue that the food is good. In addition, hospitals are notorious for being a good place to acquire an infection. While you may feel a bit overwhelmed at the prospect of going it on your own, you really don't need to remain hospitalized if there are no specific health concerns.

## Ideal Birth Worksheet

This exercise will help you sort out your thoughts and wishes about your upcoming birth. For this exercise, imagine you are having your perfect labor—everything works out exactly how you want it to.

### The Uncontrollable Issues

In real life, you cannot control these things, but if you could how would your labor happen?

- When and where does labor begin?


- Who is with you when labor begins?


- How strong are your contractions?


- How quickly do your contractions progress?


- How long do you push?



### The Almost-Controllable Issues

There are some circumstances in labor which you might have control over or might not. It all depends on how your labor unfolds. If you have a choice about these issues, how do they happen?

- How does your midwife assist you?


- Where do you labor?


- Where do you give birth?


- What tools do you use to cope with labor?

- Who labors with you?

- What techniques are used to help you?

- What techniques are not a part of your labor?

- What happens after the baby is born?

## The Most Important Issues

After working through the previous two lists of questions, you should begin to have identified the issues that are most important to you. Complete these sentences.

- My top three priorities for this birth are…

- For me, the ideal place to give birth is …

- I want to be sure that the following labor tools are available at my birth …

- For my birth, the ideal clinical personnel are …

- I want to have the following people there for my emotional support and well-being …

- For me, the best approach to pain relief is …

- The following are also very important to me …

# Birth Plan Checklist

Use this checklist to make sure you have covered everything you feel is important in your birth plan. You do not need to have something written for all these areas, this is only a list of areas you *may* have strong preferences about.

- Important Issues
    - Concerns (Why? Tell your story, briefly)
    - Health Issues
    - Fears
- Pain Management Preferences
    - 1$^{st}$ stage medications
    - Epidural
    - Water immersion
    - Non-drug comfort measures
    - Consider requesting that staff refrain from offering pain meds or asking you to rate your pain if you are attempting a natural birth
- Medical interventions you wish to use or avoid
    - For inducing or speeding up labor
    - For pain management
    - For monitoring
    - Routine administration of Pitocin for third stage (a.k.a. "active management")
- 2$^{nd}$ Stage
    - Positions you are willing/wishing to try
    - Style of pushing
    - Preferences for perineal support
- Preferences in case of cesarean
    - Type of cut on uterus (low transverse vs. vertical)
    - Who should remain with mother/baby
    - Skin-to-skin with baby as soon as possible
- Postpartum care of baby
    - Immediate undisturbed skin-to-skin with baby?
    - Delay cutting the cord until it stops pulsing?
    - Timing of routine assessments (e.g., weighing, measuring, newborn exam, etc.)
    - Routine medical interventions (e.g., Vitamin K, eye prophylaxis)?
    - Breastfeeding?
    - Rooming in or baby to nursery?
    - First bath
    - Intact penis or circumcision?
    - Consent to Hepatitis B vaccine or no?
- Other Important Items
    - Identification of support team
    - Photos/videos
    - Privacy needs
    - Environmental issues (lighting, music)

o   When to discharge
o   Educational needs (anything you want to be sure to learn about baby care before you leave)


## Sources

*Written by Patty Brennan; partially adapted from:*

- *Jennifer Vanderlaan, http://www.birthingnaturally.net/birthplan/what.html. Check out this helpful site for a variety of birth plan templates, sample birth plans, and related resources.*
- *http://www.childbirth.org/interactive/ibirthplan.html*
- *http://www.fensende.com/~swnymph/birthplan.all.html*

# Postpartum Topics

# Postpartum MotherBaby Care

Following are some things you should be watching for over the first 24 hours and early days postpartum.

## Mother

### Bleeding

Pay attention to how much you are bleeding. When you have been lying flat for any period of time, blood from your uterus will pool in the vagina. Upon rising, you will most likely feel a small gush of blood soaking your pad. This is normal. However, if you continue to bleed actively, it means that your uterus has stopped contracting. To get it contracting again, nurse your baby. You can also apply firm pressure to the uterus. Lie on your back and place the flat of your hand (or your partner's hand) on your belly, between the pubic bone and your navel. Rub firmly and deeply in a circular motion. As you do so, you will feel your uterus coming into a ball under your hand. It will be about the size of a grapefruit. (Your nurse or midwife can you show you how to do this.) Keep nursing and it should stay contracted. Check for firmness from time to time, especially the first day or two. If you are soaking a sanitary pad every thirty minutes or less, and these measures do not bring it under control, or if you are compromised from blood loss (i.e. feeling light headed, passing out), then you are bleeding too much. Call your doctor or midwife.

You may notice a blood clot or two falling into the toilet when you pee. It's good that the uterus works those out, otherwise they can contribute to extra bleeding. Passing clots may be accompanied by uterine cramping as the uterus works a little harder to contract around the clots and push them out. If you are concerned about the size or quantity of clots that you are passing, call your doctor or midwife.

### Fluids

You should have something to drink within easy reach over the next few days. Partners can help with this. Mom needs sufficient fluids to create a healthy milk supply and to flush systemic fluids, no longer needed to support the pregnancy, from her system. Extra fluids may also be present due to administration of IV fluids in labor. Water, Pregnancy Tea and juice are all good choices. Every time you sit down to nurse your baby, just make it a habit to have a drink with you.

### Urinating and Bowel Movements

It is important to keep your bladder empty after the birth. A full bladder will displace your uterus and possibly keep it from contracting properly, thereby contributing to extra bleeding. A small plastic squeeze bottle (peri bottle) will be provided at the birth center or hospital or included in your homebirth kit. Use it to rinse your perineum, in place of toilet paper, and then pat (rather than wipe) yourself dry. If you feel burning and stinging when you pee, you probably have a tear on your bottom. Fill the peri bottle up with warm water before you pee and squirt it over your perineum while you are peeing. This will dilute the urine and decrease discomfort.

Over the first few days, you may notice that you are urinating large quantities rather frequently. This is just the body dumping those extra systemic fluids. Most women find that they are also sweating, sometimes alarming quantities, soaking nightgowns and bed sheets. Not to worry … just think of it as losing a couple of pounds the easy way. Keep up your intake of fluids and the body will get the right message—to eliminate these unneeded fluids rather than hold on to them.

It is not uncommon after giving birth to feel as though you don't want to push anything else out of your body for a while. Sometimes women will get constipated postpartum because of this concern. Post-cesarean moms may also have this challenge, due to the constipating effects of narcotic pain relievers. You may want to have some prophylactic prunes or prune juice, or whatever has worked for you in the past as a natural stool softener. If you keep things soft and moving, it really won't hurt at all, despite your fears.

## Afterpains and Discomforts

After each baby, the uterus seems to have to work a little harder to stay contracted. Afterpains can be quite intense for some women after a second or third baby. Most women barely notice post-birth contractions after a first baby. As Tylenol and other pain medications create a burden for your newborn's liver, extensive use is best avoided. Homeopathics and herbs will speed the healing process as well as relieve the discomfort. The following should be available at your local health food store or online.

*Arnica 30C*
Take one dose (3–5 pellets) every three hours during the first twenty-four hours postpartum. Continue dosing three times per day for a couple of additional days. Arnica will help alleviate muscle soreness, is especially wonderful for healing vaginal bruising or a sore perineum, and also is a great post-surgical healing agent. Arnica (and, indeed, all homeopathics) can be taken concurrently with other pain-relieving medications and will not interact with them. It may enable the mother to wean off such medications more quickly.

*Magnesium Phosphate 6X*
2–3 pellets can be dissolved in ½ cup of hot water. Prepare this before you begin to nurse your baby and sip on it as needed while nursing, if afterpains are uncomfortable.

*Fema-Gen*
This herbal blend comes in capsule form. It is especially recommended for women who have had difficulty with afterpains from a previous birth or for women expecting twins or multiples.

Have it on hand for the birth. Begin with 3 doses (one dose = 2 pills) hourly after the birth x3. Repeat as needed over the first 2–3 days, gradually weaning until no longer needed.

## Most Common Big Mistake New Parents Make

*Too much company over the first few days!* It is understandable that you will feel proud of your baby and want to share him/her with family and friends. But a constant stream of visitors will interfere with establishing the breastfeeding relationship and getting much needed rest. You will need to sleep when the baby sleeps and this is likely to be very unpredictable for a while. The more you rest, the quicker you will recover. Visitors should stay briefly and be asked to contribute in some way (run an errand on their way over, bring a meal, throw in a load of laundry, change those sheets for you, etc.). Folks who have never had a baby themselves won't "get it." You will need to be explicit about your needs. Try to come up with a plan for controlling the flow of visitors and communicate it clearly. You don't want to be planning your sleep around scheduled visitors—it will be enough to have it dictated by the baby's needs.

# Baby

## Nursing

Your baby will most likely sleep once you are all settled. Many babies sleep for a good stretch right after the birth, anywhere from three to six hours, or so. This is your best opportunity for a nice recovery sleep. My advice is to turn the ringer on your phone off, delay visitors and go for it. Have your nurse put a "Sleeping—do not disturb" sign on your door. It won't stop interruptions altogether, but it will cause some folks to think twice before barging in. Over the next few weeks, your baby may want to nurse as often as every hour or two, occasionally going for longer stretches, and gradually sleeping more at night. So sleep when you can!

Nurse your baby frequently whenever he/she is awake. If the baby seems fussy or is rooting around, nurse. This will help your milk to come in quickly and then your baby may stay content for longer periods of time. If your baby just wants to sleep and sleep, or only latches on for a minute or two at a time and then falls asleep at the breast, you may need to wake the baby up to nurse. Try a bath or a diaper change to stimulate the baby and keep trying.

## Lungs

Sometimes during the first day or two, babies have some mucous they need to clear out. Usually they clear it effectively on their own, through sneezing. Occasionally, a baby may bring up some mucous which lodges in the back of the throat. They may gag on it, or you may hear it rattling there. (Stay calm—this is not life-threatening.) Simply hold the baby face down, with their chest lower than their head. You can pat their back a bit and/or use a bulb syringe to suction the mucous out if necessary. When using a bulb syringe, be sure and squeeze all the air

111

out of it before inserting it in the baby's mouth. Release your pressure once the syringe is in place and it should suck that stuff out. Remove the syringe from the baby's mouth, empty it on a diaper or whatever is handy, and repeat the process as needed. (This is rarely necessary, by the way.)

You won't be left alone after your birth until your attendants are confident that both you and the baby are stable. Some babies' lungs sound a bit rattley, while all their other vital signs are good. Babies' respirations are normally uneven. They may not take a breath for a few seconds and then take three or more quick ones in a row (30 to 50 breaths per minute is normal). Persistent fast respirations indicate that the baby is working too hard to circulate oxygen in the bloodstream and may also be a symptom of infection. If the baby's color is nice and pink all over and they are nursing, it's probably fine. A baby who is working too hard to breathe and circulate oxygen is not likely to have the extra energy to nurse.

## Cord Stump

When you change your baby's diaper, keep an eye on the cord stump over the first 24 hours. There should not be active, bright red bleeding from the stump. Over the next few days, the cord stump will rot and fall off. It may smell a little funky while this is happening, but that is normal and is not a sign of infection. However, if the skin around the base of the stump is red and puffy, or there is any discharge, then the baby's umbilicus may be infected. This is rare, but can happen. While the cord is drying up, allow as much air as possible to get at it, keeping it outside of the diaper. Recent research has shown that the best "treatment" for the cord is to do nothing. Application of rubbing alcohol to the stump was never an evidence-based practice, though it was commonly recommended.

## Urine and Meconium

Most babies will pee and pass meconium in the first 24 hours of life. It's a good idea to pay attention to this and make sure that the baby has been peeing and passing meconium. If helpers are changing diapers for you, ask them to pay attention too. Meconium is a very sticky substance and is often hard to clean off the baby's bottom. Applying a little bit of olive or vitamin E oil on the baby's bottom will make the cleanup easier. Over the first few days of life the color of the baby's poop will change, eventually turning into yellow breastfed baby poop.

# Postpartum Herbal Healing Bath

The postpartum herbal bath is wonderfully healing for both mom and baby. The recommended herbs have astringent and antiseptic properties which soothe and heal sore bottoms, help dry up the baby's cord stump and prevent infections. You and your baby can take a minimum of one bath per day for the first five days postpartum. If you have stitches or any lacerations, you may want to take two baths per day for two to three weeks, or until healing is complete. Hydrotherapy on its own is widely recommended for pain relief and healing. Add the herbs and you speed the healing process! Plus it smells good (unless you are not a fan of Lavender, in which case, just leave that herb out of the mix).

**Caution:** If you are post-surgery, then follow your doctor's recommendations regarding how long to wait before immersing the incision site in water.

## Ingredients
Calendula flowers
Comfrey leaves
Lavender flowers

## Directions
Boil a gallon of water or just use a large stock pot (it is not necessary to measure the water). Once the water boils, turn off the heat and add the contents of one pre-mixed bath to the pot. Cover and let steep for at least one hour (longer is better). When ready, pour the herb water through a strainer directly into the bath water. Discard the herbs. The mixture can sit at room temperature for up to 24 hours. If not used within 24 hours, strain out the herbs and refrigerate the fluid. It will keep for 2–3 days in the fridge. You can brew up the next batch just after the current bath is finished. Then, whenever you're ready for your next bath, it's ready for you.

As you are running the bath, keep the bathroom door closed so as to keep the room warm for the baby. Try gathering a few candles for subdued lighting which encourages the baby to open his/her eyes and overall makes for a lovely experience.

It's a good idea to have a helper if you are bringing your baby into the bath. Mom can get in first while the bath is hot and then bring baby in once it cools down a bit. Most newborns love the bath but will startle when first brought in. Have your helper hand the baby to mom and simply support the baby's head with both hands, allowing the body to immerse and float between your legs. Try to let as much of the baby be under water as possible so he/she doesn't get cold. Watch your baby relax and unfold as he/she settles in. Relax and enjoy!

You will find that the bath brings good pain relief that lasts for a period of time afterwards. Feel free to take as many as you like, with or without the herbs. You can also use a sitz bath (often supplied by the hospital or available at your local pharmacy). These just sit on the toilet (especially helpful if you don't have a tub at home) and offer a swirling stream of hot water for your bottom to soak in from a hanging plastic bag connected to the bath by a narrow plastic tube. These work really well and save you from having to get undressed and wet all over each time you would like a soak.

# Breastfeeding Primer
### By Barbara Robertson, MA, IBCLC
### The Breastfeeding Center of Ann Arbor, www.bfcaa.com


## Benefits of Breastfeeding

- Breast milk was designed to feed human babies. It is the perfect food for your baby.

- Antibodies in breast milk protect the baby from illness; lower incidence of ear infections, colic and gastro-intestinal illness.

- Breastfeeding is associated with a lower incidence of sudden infant death syndrome (SIDS).

- Breastfed babies have a decreased likelihood for allergies, dental caries and obesity.

- Breastfeeding promotes appropriate jaw, teeth and speech development, as well as overall facial development.

- Breastfeeding promotes attachment and bonding between mother and baby.

- Breastfeeding improves IQ scores in children.

- Breastfeeding helps the mother to recover from birth.
    - Promotes normal contraction and involution of the uterus, helping it to return to its pre-pregnancy size and position in the pelvis
    - Aids in postpartum weight loss
    - Contributes to normal hormonal increases and decreases associated with post-birth emotional and physical health.

- Breast milk offers your baby less exposure to pesticides, bovine growth hormone and antibiotics inherent in non-organic, commercially-produced milk used to make formula.

- Breast milk offers your baby less exposure to corn derivatives used in the production of formula and allows you to have control over the food that goes into making your baby's milk.

- Soy-based formulas can act as hormone mimics and interfere with normal hormone levels and actions in the body, affecting proper sex-differentiated development (see article at www.mothering.com, "Whole Soy Story: The Dark Side of America's Favorite Health Food" (Kaayla T. Daniel, *Mothering Magazine* Issue 124: May/June 2004).

## Comfortable Nursing

- Set up a nursing station:
    - Make a couple of comfortable places in your house to nurse, one that is private, one that is more in the center of things.
    - Ideally it would be a comfy chair that rocks, but any comfy chair, couch or bed will work.
    - Table nearby, within easy reach
    - Foot stool to prop up feet if needed
    - Try to just lay back, scoot your bottom out, tuck your tail bone under, and get comfy yourself. During feeds try and have baby's body rest on your body (see Biological Nurturing website [www.BiologicalNuturing.com] for more information.

- Make sure water and a snack are available while breastfeeding.

- Entertain yourself:
    - You'll spend a lot of time nursing in the first weeks, so make it enjoyable.
    - Develop an easy nursing activity that you love and look forward to.
    - Watch TV, read, listen to radio programs or music on an Ipod …
    - Make a place for your laptop on a nearby table and perfect your one-handed typing.
    - Engage in any activity that helps you lose yourself and keep from watching the clock.

- Nursing to sleep at night:
    - Get comfy! The side lying or laid back positions are often best when you are tired.
    - Set up a low light near the place that you will nurse to sleep at night so that you can read.
    - Use your IPod with headphones while nursing to sleep.

## Signs of Breastfeeding Trouble

### Inadequate milk supply
- Be confident in your ability to produce enough milk (most moms can) but watch for signs of inadequate intake:
    - Not enough wet diapers (less than 6–8 per day)
    - Not enough poopy diapers (less than 4 quarters worth per day)
    - Not gaining weight well (a minimum of 4 oz. per week after birth weight has been regained by day 10 or so)
    - Baby is often fussy or dissatisfied on the breast or right after a feeding.

**Engorged/Sore Breasts**
- If associated with the milk "coming in," not to worry, this will resolve on its own shortly; give the baby frequent access; if super uncomfortable, try pumping a bit off to soften your breasts to a more tolerable level; your body will automatically regulate the milk supply.
- Fresh green cabbage leaves, when applied directly to the breasts as a compress, also help to relieve discomfort. Once the leaves have wilted, replace with fresh leaves until relieved.
- Try eating a lot of watermelon and cucumbers. Both are diuretics and will help your body clear excess fluids. Moms who received IV fluids over a period of many hours during labor may have lots of edema, especially noticeable in the ankles and face, but also adding to the swollen breast tissue. The solution is simple and delicious.
- Could indicate a change in nursing frequency
- May be normal change in baby's nutritional needs
- May indicate a problem (watch for other signs of illness or concerning changes in baby)
- May be a plugged duct or the first sign of mastitis
- Go right to bed with the baby
- Extra nursing
- Lots of rest
- Drink extra water
- Massage breasts, especially while nursing
- Place a warm compress on sore area of breast
- Take warm showers or baths
- Avoid taking antibiotics unless full blown mastitis develops and does not improve with rest/nursing/hydration (could lead to thrush)

**Cracked or Sore Nipples**
- Baby is most likely having trouble with latch.
- Get some help!

**Early intervention is key when experiencing nursing trouble.**
- Call your local La Leche League leader/group
- Hire a lactation consultant, preferably one with the credentials IBCLC (International Board Certified Lactation Consultant)
- Work with a breastfeeding-friendly physician

# Breastfeeding—A Postpartum Guide

## Is my baby getting enough?

New mothers are typically concerned about whether their milk supply is sufficient. You will know if the baby is getting enough calories by counting daily stools and wet diapers. Within the first 24–48 hours the baby will pass his first stool, called meconium, which is dark and tarry. By days three to six, the baby should have two to five yellow seedy stools in a 24-hour period.

During the first two to four days, babies wet only a couple times per day. By day five or six, as mother's milk becomes more plentiful, a baby should have six to eight wet diapers in a 24-hour period. Urine should be relatively odorless and clear to pale yellow in color.

Signs of dehydration in infants include: lethargy; a sunken soft spot (anterior fontanel) on the baby's skull; dry, loose skin; diminished or absent wet diapers with concentrated urine or orange staining due to uric acid crystals; dry mucous membranes (look in the baby's mouth—are saliva bubbles visible?); temperature; and fast respirations (persistently greater than 30–50 breaths per minute). (These last two symptoms may also indicate infection in the newborn, which is an emergency.)

## How often and how long should I nurse?

Women are often surprised to discover that it is normal for an exclusively breastfed infant to nurse every 1½ hours in the first couple of weeks. Feeding may last 30 minutes to one hour. Frequent feeding promotes adequate weight gain. Furthermore, milk production follows the principle of "supply and demand." Nursing at least 8–15 times every 24 hours will assure a sufficient milk supply to meet the baby's needs.

Remember: Feedings are variable in duration and intensity during the early weeks. The ZEN of breastfeeding is to "watch the baby, not the clock." Check for adequate wets and stools. It is the frequency of breastfeeding rather than the duration that actually stimulates milk production.

## Weight gain

Initially babies typically lose up to 10 percent of their birth weight. By day three to five, the baby will begin gaining about ½ to 1 ounce per day. Babies should regain their birth weight by day 10. After day 10, babies should be gaining a minimum of 4 ounces per week. If infants follow this pattern, you can feel confident that they are getting enough milk.

Be aware that weighing the baby on different scales (such as one at the hospital, one at home, and one at the pediatrician's office) is likely to yield slight differences in calibration which do not reflect a failure-to-thrive or insufficient milk supply problem. Weighing the baby too frequently (daily or more than once per day) should be discouraged. Trust your eyes and intuition as well.

# Still Eating for Two—Nourishing the Breastfeeding Mother
## By Barbara Robertson, MA, IBCLC

Excerpted from our cookbook,
*Whole Family Recipes: For the Childbearing Year & Beyond*
Edited by Patty Brennan, www.center4cby.com

Sadly, some mothers quit nursing because they feel their diets are inadequate or they have to eat special foods. Many cultures have rules about what you should or should not eat, but little of what passes for advice has been substantiated by research. Even if a mom's milk might be a bit deficient, it still beats artificial human milk (formula) by far. Throughout my eleven years of breastfeeding I heard a lot of advice about what to eat and what to avoid while nursing. Myths abound on the subject. As a professional lactation consultant, I have looked into the research on this subject. Here are some things I have learned about maternal nutrition and breastfeeding.

## Common Myths

*You have to eat a special diet or your milk won't be good enough.* False! The mother's body will take what it needs to make milk, perhaps depleting the mother's stores of nutrients. The mother might become malnourished, but the baby will be fine. Mothers in third-world countries who are mildly to moderately malnourished are nevertheless able to produce an adequate supply of good quality milk. Only under famine or near-famine conditions is the supply or composition of breast milk compromised. There are a few foods that can improve the quality of breast milk and a few substances that can make breast milk less nutritious, but, in general, moms can eat what they like and still make good milk. On the other hand, moms will feel better and be healthier if they eat a well-balanced, whole foods diet.

*You have to drink cow's milk to make human milk.* False! This I have personal experience with. For most of my life, I avoided drinking cow's milk due to being lactose intolerant. While I was pregnant with my son, I craved it and began drinking it. After he was born, I continued to drink it because of this myth. However, my digestive system protested my behavior. When I eliminated the cow's milk products, all of my symptoms went away and my milk production was fine.

*Foods that make you gassy such as beans, broccoli, cabbage and cauliflower will make your baby gassy.* False! Sometimes a baby might be sensitive to something in your diet, but it's usually not one of these foods. What makes these foods gassy is how the structure of the complex carbohydrates and high-fiber foods reacts with the digestive tract. By the time this food is transformed into breast milk the gas-producing factors are no longer an issue.

119

*Vegetarian and vegan moms don't produce adequate milk.* False! They need to supplement with vitamins B6 and B12, but as long as they are eating well, their milk will be fine.

*You cannot eat chocolate or drink caffeine or alcohol.* False! Most babies do not react at all with moderate consumption of these substances. Moderation seems to be the key here.

*A mom can't diet while breastfeeding.* False! It is recommended that a mother go no lower than 1,800 calories a day and lose no more than 1 pound a week while breastfeeding, but this is good advice for all people who want to lose weight, not just breastfeeding moms.


## Some Things I Have Found to Be True

*Nursing mothers are hungry mothers.* You need an extra 300–500 calories per day, over and above your pregnancy diet, to make milk. We encourage moms to eat nutritiously and to eat when hungry, rather than becoming fanatical about counting calories.

*Nursing mothers are thirsty mothers.* We know that fluids are good for us, but nursing moms are especially thirsty. Once again, we encourage moms to drink to thirst. Some moms drink too much water, which can lower milk production and affect electrolyte balance in the body. We encourage every mom to have a glass of water nearby when she sits to nurse the baby.

*Breast milk changes flavor depending on what you eat.* This is a good thing! Breastfed babies have an easier time switching to solids and eating a wide variety of foods compared to formula-fed babies. Imagine having eaten nothing but one uninspired (have you ever tasted formula?) food for six months. It's hard to adjust. Breast milk can also change color (although it usually doesn't) with what you eat or drink. Apparently, foods or drinks with large quantities of dyes can stain breast milk and/or the baby's urine.

*Dairy products.* If a baby has mucus and/or blood in his/her stools, consider eliminating cow's milk products from mom's diet. In several studies, about half of the babies' stools improved quickly when moms eliminated dairy from their diets.

*Some foods can reduce the mother's milk supply.* Possible culprits are sage, mint and parsley, so you may want to avoid your stuffing and tabouli while nursing. On the other hand, a mom who needs to dry up her milk supply (for whatever reason) can brew up three strong cups of sage tea per day (3 teaspoons dried sage to 3 cups boiled water, covered and steeped for at least 2 hours). Take until the milk is gone, slowly weaning off the tea so as to avoid a rebound effect.

*The fats a mother eats affect the types of fats present in her breast milk.* Essential fatty acids (EFAs) are found in nuts, seeds, fish, and greens and are passed from mom to baby. EFAs are converted into arachidonic acid (AA), eicosapentaenoic acid (EPA), and docosahexaenoic acid (DHA). We know that AA and DHA are important for brain development. Trans-fatty acids (TFAs) are also passed to the baby. These are not good for mom or baby. So it's important to monitor what kinds of fats are in your diet. If a mom cuts back on her TFA intake or adds more EFAs, the milk will adjust in a few days to these positive changes.

This is something we think might be true; we've seen it in practice, but it hasn't been studied in detail yet. Adding healthy fats to the mother's diet appears to be related to improved milk quality or production—we are not sure which. After a few weeks, a mom will go from having a fussy baby to having a satisfied baby. Is it because there are more calories (cream) in the milk, or is she just making more of it? Some of these healthy fats are coconut, avocado, nuts and seeds, butter, olive oil and foods high in omega threes. She should try and eat the foods rather than taking supplements, but supplements are better than nothing. Think guacamole, salmon, coconut macaroons …

*You can help prevent known family allergies by not eating trigger foods while nursing.* This is true for nuts and other offenders. Some pediatricians recommend that all mothers avoid nuts while nursing.

*Contaminated breast milk.* Nursing mothers (perhaps all mothers) should avoid eating fish high in mercury such as shark, swordfish, king mackerel and tilefish. The mercury can be passed from mother to baby in breast milk. However, even contaminated milk is healthier than formula in almost all cases.

*Worried about your milk supply?* Adding a bowl of oatmeal a day to your diet can help! There seem to be trace nutrients in whole grains that help with milk production, and the less processed, the better.

# Choosing a Pediatrician

**Do we need a pediatrician?**

Pediatricians specialize in helping sick babies. If your baby is healthy and you have a family practice doctor with whom you are comfortable, you may not need a private pediatrician for your baby. To read an insider's account critical of the practice of "well baby visits," see Robert Mendelsohn's book, *How to Raise a Healthy Child in Spite of Your Doctor.* In my opinion, this book picks up where most childbirth preparation classes leave off—with a consumer approach to medical care for infants and children.

If your family has a preference for a specific type of complementary medicine, for example, a family doctor who specializes in homeopathic medicine, then it might make more sense to simply stick with your family practice physician to handle care for the whole family.

On the other hand, if your comfort level is more in sync with current allopathic medical practice, then it can be a good idea to identify a pediatrician with whom you feel comfortable prior to your baby's birth. That way, you have someone who can provide immediate follow up after the birth and, if your baby is born with any medical issues, a second opinion from a trusted source is immediately available to you.

See our Additional Resources / Best of the Web for a link to a helpful article.

# Newborn Babies and Sleep
## Excerpted with permission by Elizabeth Pantley, Author of
### *The No-Cry Sleep Solution* and *Gentle Baby Care*
### www.pantley.com

Congratulations on the birth of your new baby. This is a glorious time in your life—and a sleepless time too. Newborns have very different sleep needs than older babies. This article will help you understand your baby's developing sleep patterns and will help you have reasonable expectations for sleep.

### Read, Learn and Beware of Bad Advice

Absolutely *everyone* has an opinion about how you should handle sleep issues with your new baby. The danger to a new parent is that these tidbits of misguided advice (no matter how well intentioned) can truly have a negative effect on our parenting skills and, by extension, our babies' development ... *if we are not aware of the facts*. The more knowledge you have the less likely that other people will make you doubt your parenting decisions. When you have your facts straight, and when you have a parenting plan, you will be able to respond with confidence to those who are well-meaning but offering contrary or incorrect advice. So, your first step is to get smart! Know *what* you are doing, and know *why* you are doing it. Read books and magazines, attend classes or support groups—it all helps.

### The Biology of Newborn Sleep

During the early months of your baby's life, he sleeps when he is tired, it's that simple. You can do little to force a new baby to sleep when he doesn't want to sleep, and conversely, you can do little to wake him up when he is sleeping soundly. Newborn babies have very tiny tummies. They grow rapidly, their diet is liquid and it digests quickly. Although it would be nice to lay your little bundle down at bedtime and not hear from him until morning, this is not a realistic goal for a tiny baby. Newborns need to be fed every two to four hours—and often more frequently.

### Sleeping "Through the Night"

You may believe that babies should start "sleeping through the night" soon after birth. For a new baby, *a five-hour stretch* is a full night. Many (but not all) babies *can* sleep uninterrupted from midnight to 5 a.m. (Not that they always do.) This may be a far cry from what you may have thought "sleeping through the night" meant! What's more, some sleep-through-the-nighters will suddenly begin waking more frequently and it's often a full year, or even two, until your baby will settle into an all-night, every-night sleep pattern.

### Falling Asleep at the Breast or Bottle

It is natural for a newborn to fall asleep while sucking at the breast, a bottle or a pacifier. When a baby *always* falls asleep this way, he learns to associate sucking with falling asleep; over time, he cannot fall asleep any other way. This is probably the most natural, pleasant sleep association a baby can have. However, a large percentage of parents who are struggling with older babies who cannot fall asleep or stay asleep are fighting this powerful association. Therefore, if you want your baby to be able to fall asleep without your help, it is essential that you *sometimes* let your newborn baby suck until he is sleepy, but not totally asleep. When you can, remove the breast, bottle or pacifier from his mouth and let him finish falling asleep without it. If you do this often enough, he will learn how to fall asleep without sucking.

## Waking for Night Feedings

Many pediatricians recommend that parents shouldn't let a newborn sleep longer than four hours without feeding and the majority of babies wake far more frequently than that. No matter what, your baby *will* wake up during the night. The key is to learn when you should pick her up for a feeding and when you can let her go back to sleep on her own. Here's a tip that is important for you to know. Babies make many sleeping sounds, from grunts to whimpers to outright cries and these noises don't always signal awakening. These are what I call *sleeping noises* and your baby is asleep during these episodes. Learn to differentiate between sleeping sounds and awake sounds. If she is awake and hungry, you'll want to feed her as quickly as possible so she'll go back to sleep easily. But if she's asleep—let her sleep!

## Help Your Baby Distinguish Day from Night

A newborn sleeps sixteen to eighteen hours per day and this sleep is distributed evenly over six to seven sleep periods. You can help your baby distinguish between night sleep and day sleep, and thus help him sleep longer periods at night. Have your baby take his daytime naps in a lit room where he can hear the noises of the day. Make nighttime sleep dark and quiet, except for white noise (a background hum). You can also help your baby differentiate day from night by using a nightly bath and a change into pajamas (or other ritual) to signal the difference between the two.

## Watch for Signs of Tiredness

Get familiar with your baby's sleepy signals and put her down to sleep as soon as she seems tired. A baby who is encouraged to stay awake when her body is craving sleep is an unhappy baby. Over time, this pattern develops into sleep deprivation, which complicates developing sleep maturity. Learn to read your baby's sleepy signs—such as quieting down, losing interest in people and toys, and fussing—and put her to bed when that window of opportunity presents itself.

## Make Yourself Comfortable

It's a fact that your baby *will* be waking you up, so you may as well make yourself as comfortable as possible. Relax about night waking right now. Being frustrated about having to get up won't change a thing. The situation will improve day by day. Before you know it, your newborn won't be so little anymore—she'll be walking and talking and getting into everything in sight during the day and sleeping peacefully all night long.

# Infant Sleep Environment Safety Checklist

## Recommendations that apply to infant sleep in both cribs and adult beds

- Use a firm mattress. A soft mattress can result in infant suffocation.

- There should be no gaps between the mattress and the frame of the crib or bed. Infants and small children can become wedged in gaps and asphyxiate.

- Bedding should fit tightly around the mattress. Fitted sheets that become loose from a corner can cover and smother a baby.

- Avoid strings or ties on all nightclothes (both baby's and parents'). These pose a strangulation risk.

- Avoid soft bedding and other items, including comforters, pillows, featherbeds, stuffed animals, lamb skins, bean bags, etc. Bumper pads should not be used. Each of these poses a risk of suffocation.

- Keep baby's face uncovered to allow ventilation.

- Put baby on his or her back to sleep. Babies sleeping on their backs are less likely to become victims of sudden infant death syndrome (SIDS).

- Adults should avoid smoking. Exposure to tobacco, both pre- and post-delivery, is associated with a higher risk of SIDS.

- Avoid overheating the room in which the baby sleeps and avoid overdressing the baby. Overheating is associated with an increased risk of SIDS.

- Avoid placing a crib near window treatment cords or sashes. These pose a strangulation risk.

## Advice specific to cribs

- When baby learns to sit, lower the mattress level so that he or she cannot fall out or climb over the side rail.

- When baby learns to stand, set the mattress level at its lowest point.

- When baby reaches a height of 35 inches or the side rail is less than three-quarters of his or her height, move the baby to another bed. Babies can fall from their cribs if the side rails are not at the right level in relationship to the mattress surface.

- Hang crib mobiles well out of reach and remove them when baby starts to sit or reaches five months of age, whichever comes first. Mobiles become strangulation or choking hazards if baby can reach them.

- Remove crib gyms when baby can get up on all fours. Babies can become entangled in these and risk strangulation.

- Keep baby warm by dressing him or her in a blanket sleeper or "sleep sack."

## General advice regarding infant sleep

- Do not sleep with baby on sofas or overstuffed chairs.

- Do not place baby (particularly one born prematurely) to sleep in car or infant seats as these can fail to adequately support the infant's upper body, block the baby's airway and put baby at risk for suffocation.

- Parents who choose to bed share with their infants must be proactive. They must evaluate their sleep environment and make it as safe as possible for their baby. Both parents should feel comfortable with the decision to place baby in the environment that is chosen, whether crib or adult bed, and should be committed to following that environment's safety precautions, as noted above. No one sleep environment can guarantee that a baby will be risk free, but there are ways of reducing risk in both cribs and adult beds.

## Risk factors for bed-sharing

- Very small premature or low birth-weight babies appear to be at greater risk when bed-sharing, but benefit greatly from co-sleeping nearby but on a separate surface.

- Do not sleep with baby if you are currently a smoker or if you smoked during pregnancy.

- Do not sleep on the same surface as your baby if you are overly tired or have ingested alcohol/sedatives/drugs (or any substance that makes you less aware).

- Baby appears to be safest when sleeping beside his/her breastfeeding mother.

- Older siblings or other children should not sleep with babies under one year old.

- Do not swaddle your baby when bed-sharing. Baby may overheat (which is a risk factor for SIDS) and a swaddled baby is not able to effectively move covers from the face or use arms and legs to alert an adult.

- Other potential hazards: very long hair should be tied up so that it does not become wrapped around baby's neck; a parent who is an exceptionally deep sleeper or an extremely obese parent who has a problem feeling exactly how close baby is should consider having baby sleep nearby, but on a separate sleep surface.

# Postpartum Planning Guide

These are guidelines for the first few weeks following an uneventful birth. In the case of twins, prolonged or difficult labor and birth, cesarean delivery, maternal hemorrhage, severe perineal lacerations, or health issues with the baby requiring extended hospitalization, your plan should allow extra time for care and recovery.

*Hint: After the baby is born, pull out this guide and re-read it!*

1.  **Plan for household help.** Recruit the support of one or two mentally positive people to free the mother of household responsibilities (laundry, shopping, errands, cleaning, meal preparation, child care for older siblings) for two to six weeks. Your support folks should be able to see what needs doing and do it without lots of direction. There is to be no guilt involved with asking for help! If extended family support is available to you, that can work or, if you can afford it, consider hiring a postpartum doula. To learn more about the role of postpartum doulas, see the article "All about Doulas: A Consumers' Guide to Getting the Help You Need" at www.center4cby.com.

2.  **Control visitors.** Inform close friends and family when you are ready for visitors after birth. It is important to control who, when, how many at a time, and for how long you want to welcome visitors. You will, no doubt, be eager to show off your baby. On the other hand, visitors arriving just as you have an opportunity to sleep, or when you should be focusing on breastfeeding your baby, will likely prove to be more stressful than enjoyable. Turn the ringer off your phone to sleep. Post signs saying "We are sleeping now. Please come another time." Plan for short visits and ask guests to bring food or help with chores. Remember that people who have never had a baby before will be relatively clueless as to your needs. You will need to clue them in. Failure to control the number and timing of visitors is probably the most common mistake new parents make.

3.  **Sleep when the baby sleeps.** Calculate the average amount of sleep you need to feel okay under normal circumstances. Can you normally get by with six or seven hours, or do you need eight or nine to feel well? You will still need this same amount of sleep after the baby is born, though admittedly it will be interrupted sleep. One strategy is to not get up and get dressed, receive visitors, or go about your day until you actually have managed to sleep your required amount. On some days, this may be well into the afternoon hours. Resist the temptation to "do everything" when the baby is sleeping if you have not gotten your eight hours (or whatever) in during the last twenty-four hours. The more you rest now, the sooner you will recover.

4.  **Heal.** Listen to your body and take care of yourself. Milk supply and postpartum healing are your top priorities. In addition to sleeping, make sure you are drinking plenty of fluids and eating properly. Take sitz baths if you have stitches—even two or

three times per day to promote healing and control pain. Remember healing is a *process* rather than a *result.* And healing takes time.

5. **Recruit help with meals.** Make a list of things your family likes to eat. Post this list on the refrigerator for all to see. This provides a quick answer for those asking to bring a meal. It may be helpful to appoint someone to organize meals for the family. Online calendars are a great tool. When folks sign up to drop off a meal, make it easy for a meal to be left for you without necessarily having to be awake to receive the meal or invite guests in (e.g., a cooler on the porch). In addition, you may want to freeze some meals ahead of time and stock up on non-perishables. Use these when your helpers start to fade.

6. **Consider paying for help.** This may include housecleaning, childcare for your other children, using a diaper service for the first six weeks, or hiring a postpartum doula. If you can't afford to hire help, perhaps ask for help as a shower gift rather than accumulating a bunch of stuff that you don't really need.

7. **Ask for what you need**. Postpartum can be emotionally high and low all at the same time. Hormones are changing dramatically. You may just need someone to listen to you and validate your feelings about your birth, about becoming a mother, or other challenges you are experiencing. Lots of new parents are disturbed by some of the emotions they are experiencing postpartum as they go through this tremendous adjustment to parenthood. It's okay. Talk about it. You are not alone.

8. **Have realistic expectations.** Newborns "only" sleep, eat and poop, but they do it every hour (or so). It takes more time and energy than most people realize. Imagine a sphere about 1" in diameter. That's how big a newborn's tummy is! As breast milk is easily digested, it moves quickly out of the stomach and the baby is hungry again. As your baby grows, he/she will grow a bigger stomach and be able to space out their feedings a bit more. Each one is different, some sleeping five hours at a stretch from the early weeks on, and others waking every hour and a half to nurse for months. Let your baby lead the way at first. Try and keep it in perspective; things change quickly.

9. **Understand that siblings go through adjustment too.** While accepting help to care for them, try to keep established rituals intact so that your child doesn't feel abandoned or utterly displaced. If you normally read a book to your child before bedtime, then make every effort to continue to do so. It is not uncommon for toddlers to relapse with toilet training efforts when there is a new baby in the house (don't despair with this!). Consider recruiting helpers to take your child for an outing. Breastfeeding mothers of toddlers find that having a "special" basket of toys that only comes out when it's time to nurse the baby is a good strategy. Or limit video watching to only breastfeeding times, or listen to books on CD together, to be continued at the next breastfeeding session…. You can get really creative here.

10. **Take a little time for yourself each day.** At first, it can feel as though, if you are meeting the baby's needs, then your needs don't get met. It is only normal that you may feel sad or even resentful about this. Try to identify what activity you miss the most. Are you longing for a walk in fresh air, girlfriend time, computer play time, or missing your exercise regime? Try to carve out even a half hour where you and your partner give each other permission to get at least that one need met. Make a list right now of three things you find relaxing, rejuvenating or inspiring.

11. **Don't forget to take time for each other.** Many new moms experience a drop in their sex drive for a while after giving birth. This is normal, it's okay, and it will return. Breastfeeding a baby involves a great deal of intimacy and new moms may feel "touched out." A fear that sex will hurt, especially if there was trauma to the perineum or vagina, is understandable. Also your hormones are not helping out because your body is not really trying to get pregnant right now. With the ebb and flow of cycles and desire, you may find yourself solidly in the ebb for a while. For breastfeeding mothers, the hormones that promote fertility and the presence of cervical mucus remain suppressed (timing is variable on this, lasting anywhere from a few weeks postpartum through the full time that mom breastfeeds). This means that the vagina may be dryer than usual, requiring lubrication for sex to feel comfortable. There are all kinds of intimacy. A dinner by candlelight, a "date night," a walk together without the baby, or willingness to pleasure your partner without feeling you have to respond in kind are all creative solutions. Patience and mutual consideration are key.

12. **Postpone major life changes.** When possible, avoid moving or changing jobs during the childbearing year (pregnancy through at least three months postpartum). Many new parents imagine they require more space for their expanding family. Maybe you don't actually need a nursery or a bigger home or all of that baby gear. Keep it simple and play it by ear. Having a baby is change enough.

13. **Develop a support network.** Hook up with both new and experienced parents for support, guidance and feedback. In the end, this will normalize what you are experiencing OR perhaps help you determine that your situation is not normal and that you need extra help. Either way, it should prove validating.

14. **Give yourself credit.** Parenting is a huge life change, bringing more love and laughter into your life along with new challenges. The difficult times and the adoration you feel for your baby do not necessarily balance out to a happy medium. It can be both joyful and hard. It may take some time for you to find your new rhythm.

# Handling Unwanted Advice
**Excerpted with permission by Elizabeth Pantley,**
**Author of *The No-Cry Sleep Solution* and *Gentle Baby Care***
**www.pantley.com**

*"Help! I'm getting so frustrated with the endless stream of advice I get from my mother-in-law and brother! No matter what I do, I'm doing it wrong. I love them both, but how do I get them to stop dispensing all this unwanted advice?"*

Just as your baby is an important part of your life, he is also important to others. People who care about your baby are bonded to you and your child in a special way that invites their counsel. Knowing this may give you a reason to handle the interference gently, in a way that leaves everyone's feelings intact. Regardless of the advice, it is *your* baby and in the end, you will raise your child the way that you think best. So it's rarely worth creating a war over a well-meaning person's comments. You can respond to unwanted advice in a variety of ways:

### Listen first
It's natural to be defensive if you feel that someone is judging you; but chances are you are not being criticized; rather, the other person is sharing what they feel to be valuable insight. Try to listen—you may just learn something valuable.

### Disregard
If you know that there is no convincing the other person to change her mind, simply smile, nod and make a non-committal response such as, "Interesting!" Then go about your own business ... your way.

### Agree
You might find one part of the advice that you agree with. If you can, provide wholehearted agreement on that topic.

### Pick your battles
If your mother-in-law insists that baby wear a hat on your walk to the park, go ahead and pop one on his head. This won't have any long-term effects except that of placating her. However, don't capitulate on issues that are important to you or the health or well-being of your child.

### Steer clear of the topic
If your brother is pressuring you to let your baby cry to sleep, but you would never do that, then don't complain to him about your baby getting you up five times the night before. If *he* brings up the topic, then distraction is definitely in order, such as, "Would you like a cup of coffee?"

131

**Educate yourself**

Knowledge is power; protect yourself and your sanity by reading up on your parenting choices. Rely on the confidence that you are doing your best for your baby.

**Educate the other person**

If your "teacher" is imparting information that you know to be outdated or wrong, share what you've learned on the topic. You may be able to open the other person's mind. Refer to a study, book or report that you have read.

**Quote a doctor**

Many people accept a point of view if a professional has validated it. If your own pediatrician agrees with your position, say, "My doctor said to wait until she's at least six months before starting solids." If your *own* doctor doesn't back your view on that issue, then refer to another doctor—perhaps the author of a baby care book.

**Be vague**

You can avoid confrontation with an elusive response. For example, if your sister asks if you've started potty training yet (but you are many months away from even starting the process), you can answer with, "We're moving in that direction."

***Ask* for advice!**

Your friendly counselor is possibly an expert on a few issues that you can agree on. Search out these points and invite guidance. She'll be happy that she is helping you and you'll be happy you have a way to avoid a showdown about topics that you *don't* agree on.

**Memorize a standard response**

Here's a comment that can be said in response to almost any piece of advice: "This may not be the right way for you, but it's the right way for *me*."

**Be honest**

Try being honest about your feelings. Pick a time free of distractions and choose your words carefully, such as, "I know how much you love Harry and I'm glad you spend so much time with him. I know you think you're helping me when you give me advice about this, but I'm comfortable with my own approach and I'd really appreciate if you'd understand that."

**Find a mediator**

If the situation is putting a strain on your relationship with the advice-giver, you may want to ask another person to step in for you.

**Search out like-minded friends**

Join a support group or on-line club with people who share your parenting philosophies. Talking with others who are raising their babies in a way that is similar to your own can give you the strength to face people who don't understand your viewpoints.

# How to Calm Your Crying Baby
**Excerpted with permission by Elizabeth Pantley,**
**Author of *The No-Cry Sleep Solution* and *Gentle Baby Care***
**www.pantley.com**

When we're pregnant or awaiting adoption, we dream about our baby-to-be, we always envision those beautiful Hallmark card scenes: charming baby smiling up at peaceful mother's face. We read books in advance of the big day about how care for a newborn—how to bathe, feed and dress her—and then we feel somewhat prepared. However, a crying baby was never part of that idyllic vision, so this takes us by surprise. But the fact is, all babies cry at one time or another. Some babies cry more than others, but they all do cry. Understanding *why* babies cry can help you get through this phase and respond effectively to your crying baby.

## Why does my baby cry?

Simply put, babies cry because they cannot talk. Babies are human beings and they have needs and desires, just as we do, but they can't express them. Even if they could talk, very often they wouldn't understand why they feel the way they do, they wouldn't understand themselves well enough to articulate their needs, so babies need someone to help them figure it all out. Their cries are the only way they can say, "Help me! Something isn't right here!"

## Different kinds of cries

As you get to know your baby, you'll become the expert in understanding his cries in a way that no one else can. In their research, child development professionals have determined that certain types of cries mean certain things. In other words, babies don't cry the same exact way every time. (Other child development experts, also known as mothers, have known that for millennia.) Over time, you'll recognize particular cries as if they were spoken words. In addition to these cry signals, you often can determine why your baby is crying by the situation surrounding the cry. Following are common reasons for baby's cry and the clues that may tell you what's up.

**Hunger:** If two or more hours have passed since his last feeding, if he has just woken up, or if he has just had a very full diaper and he begins to cry, he's probably hungry. A feeding will most likely stop the crying.

**Tiredness:** Look for these signs: decreased activity, losing interest in people and toys, rubbing eyes, looking glazed, and the most obvious—yawning. If you notice any of these in your crying baby, she may just need to sleep. Time for bed!

**Discomfort:** If a baby is uncomfortable—too wet, hot, cold, squished—he'll typically squirm or arch his back when he cries, as if trying to get away from the source of his discomfort. Try to figure out the source of his distress and solve his problem.

**Pain:** A cry of pain is sudden and shrill, just like when an adult or older child cries out when they get hurt. It may include long cries followed by a pause during which your baby appears to stop breathing. He then catches his breath and lets out another long cry. Time to check your baby's temperature and undress him for a full-body examination.

**Overstimulation:** If the room is noisy, people are trying to get your baby's attention, rattles are rattling, music boxes are playing, and your baby suddenly closes her eyes and cries (or turns her head away), she may be trying to shut out all that's going on around her and find some peace. It's time for a quiet, dark room and some peaceful cuddles.

**Illness:** When your baby is sick, he may cry in a weak, moaning way. This is his way of saying, "I feel awful." If your baby seems ill, look for any signs of sickness, take his temperature and call your healthcare provider.

**Frustration.** Your baby is just learning how to control her hands, arms and feet. She may be trying to get her fingers into her mouth or to reach a particularly interesting toy, but her body isn't cooperating. She cries out of frustration, because she can't accomplish what she wants to do. All she needs is a little help.

**Loneliness:** If your baby falls asleep feeding and you place her in her crib, but she wakes soon afterward with a cry, she may be saying that she misses the warmth of your embrace and doesn't like to be alone. A simple situation to resolve …

**Worry or fear.** Your baby suddenly finds himself in the arms of Great Aunt Matilda and can't see you; his previously happy gurgles turn suddenly to crying. He's trying to tell you that he's scared. He doesn't know this new person and he wants Mommy or Daddy. Explain to Auntie that he needs a little time to warm up to someone new and try letting the two of them get to know each other while baby stays in your arms.

**Boredom.** Your baby has been sitting in his infant seat for 20 minutes while you talk and eat lunch with a friend. He's not tired, hungry or uncomfortable, but he starts a whiny, fussy cry. He may be saying that he's bored and needs something new to look at or touch. A new position for his seat or a toy to hold may help.

**Colic.** If your baby cries inconsolably for long periods every day, particularly at the same time each day, he may have colic. Researchers are still unsure of colic's exact cause. Some experts believe that colic is related to the immaturity of a baby's digestive system. Whatever the cause, and it may be a combination of all the theories, colic is among the most exasperating conditions that parents of new babies face. Colic occurs only to newborn babies, up to about four to five months of age. Look for patterns to your baby's crying; these can provide clues as to which suggestions are most likely to help. Then experiment with some of the ideas on the following list and in the rest of this article.

- If breastfeeding, feed on demand (cue feeding), for nutrition as well as comfort, as often as your baby needs a calming influence.
- If breastfeeding, try avoiding foods that may cause gas in your baby, such as dairy products, caffeine, cabbage, broccoli and other gassy vegetables.
- If bottle feeding, offer more frequent but smaller meals; experiment with different formulas with your doctor or health care provider's approval.
- If bottle feeding, try different types of bottles and nipples that prevent air from entering your baby as he drinks, such as those with curved bottles or collapsible liners.
- Hold your baby in a more upright position for feeding and directly afterwards.
- Experiment with how often and when you burp your baby.
- Offer meals in a quiet setting.
- If baby likes a pacifier, offer him one.
- Invest in a baby sling or carrier and use it during colicky periods.
- If the weather's too unpleasant for an outside stroll, bring your stroller in the house and walk your baby around.
- Give your baby a warm bath.
- Hold your baby with her legs curled up toward her belly.
- Massage your baby's tummy or give him a full massage.
- Swaddle your baby in a warm blanket.
- Lay your baby tummy down across your lap and massage or pat her back.
- Hold your baby in a rocking chair or put him in a swing.
- Walk with baby in a quiet, dark room while you hum or sing.
- Try keeping your baby away from highly stimulating situations during the day, when possible, to prevent sensory overload.
- Lie on your back and lay your baby on top of you, tummy down, while massaging his back. (Transfer your baby to his bed if he falls asleep.)
- Take baby for a ride in the car.
- Play soothing music or turn on white noise such as a fan.
- As a last resort, ask your doctor or health care provider about medications available for colic and gas. Alternatives such as herbal teas and homeopathy may help as well.

## What about fussy crying?

There are plenty of times when you can't tell if your baby's crying is directly related to a fixable situation: hunger, a soiled diaper or a longing to be held. That's when parents get frustrated and nervous. That's when you should take a deep breath and try some of the following cry-stoppers.

*Hold your baby.* No matter the reason for your baby's cry, being held by a warm and comforting person offers a feeling of security and may calm his crying. Babies love to be held in arms, slings, front-pack carriers and slings, and (when they get a little older) backpacks. Physical contact is what they seek and what usually soothes them best.

*Breastfeed your baby.* Nursing your baby is as much for comfort as food. All four of my babies calmed easily when brought to the breast—so much so that my husband has always called it

"The Secret Weapon." And my babies are very typical. Breastfeeding is an important and powerful tool for baby soothing.

*Provide motion*. Babies enjoy repetitive, rhythmic motion such as rocking, swinging, swaying, jiggling, dancing or a drive in the car. Many parents instinctually begin to sway with a fussy baby and for a good reason: It works.

*Turn on some white noise*. The womb was a very noisy place. Remember the sounds you heard on the Doppler stethoscope? Not so long ago, your baby heard those 24 hours a day. Therefore, your baby sometimes can be calmed by "white noise," that is, noise that is continuous and uniform, such as that of a heartbeat, the rain, static between radio stations, a fan, and so on. Some alarm clocks even have a white noise function.

*Let music soothe your baby.* Soft, peaceful music is a wonderful baby calmer. That's why lullabies have been passed down through the ages. You don't have to be a professional singer to provide your baby with a song; your baby loves to hear your voice. In addition to your own songs, babies usually love to hear any kind of music. Experiment with different types of tunes, since babies have their own favorites that can range from jazz to country to classical, and even rock and rap.

*Swaddle your baby.* During the first three or four months of life, many babies feel comforted if you can re-create the tightly contained sensation they enjoyed in the womb..

*Massage your baby.* Babies love to be touched and stroked, so a massage is a wonderful way to calm a fussy baby. A variation of massage is the baby pat; many babies love a gentle, rhythmic pat on their backs or bottoms.

*Let your baby have something to suck on.* The most natural pacifier is mother's breast, but when that isn't an option, a bottle, pacifier, baby's own fingers, a teething toy, or a pinkie can work wonders as a means of comfort.

*Distract your baby.* Sometimes a new activity or change of scenery—maybe a walk outside, or a dance with a song, or a splashy bath—can be very helpful in turning a fussy baby into a happy one.

## Reading your baby's body language

Many times, you can avoid the crying altogether by responding right away to your baby's earliest signals of need, such as fussing, stiffening her body or rooting for the breast. As you get to know your baby and learn her signals, determining what she needs will become easier for you, even before she cries.

# The T.I.C.K.S. Rule for Safe Babywearing

Keep your baby close and keep your baby safe. When you're wearing a sling or carrier, don't forget the T.I.C.K.S.

- ✓ Tight
- ✓ In view at all times
- ✓ Close enough to kiss
- ✓ Keep chin off the chest
- ✓ Supported back

**Tight:** Slings and carriers should be tight enough to hug your baby close to you as this will be most comfortable for you both. Any slack/loose fabric will allow your baby to slump down in the carrier which can hinder their breathing and pull on your back.

**In View at All Times:** You should always be able to see your baby's face by simply glancing down. The fabric of a sling or carrier should not close around them so you have to open it to check on them. In a cradle position, your baby should face upwards, not be turned in towards your body.

**Close Enough to Kiss:** Your baby's head should be as close to your chin as is comfortable. By tipping your head forward, you should be able to kiss your baby on the head or forehead.

**Keep Chin Off the Chest:** A baby should never be curled so their chin is forced onto their chest as this can restrict their breathing. Ensure there is always a space of at least a finger width under your baby's chin.

**Supported Back:** In an upright carry, a baby should be held comfortably close to the wearer so their back is supported in its natural position and their tummy and chest are against you. If a sling is too loose, they can slump, which can partially close their airway. (This can be tested by placing a hand on your baby's back and pressing gently; they should not uncurl or move closer to you.) A baby in a cradle carry in a pouch or ring sling should be positioned carefully with their bottom in the deepest part so the sling does not fold them in half, pressing their chin to their chest.

# Additional Resources

# Additional Resources

## Recommended Reading

- Brennan, Patty. *Guide to Homeopathic Remedies for the Birth Bag, 5th Edition;* www.center4cby.com.
- Brennan, Patty. *Vaccines & Informed Choice: Everything Parents Need to Know, 5th Edition;* summarizes vaccine controversies, how to prevent adverse vaccine reactions, how to enhance natural immunity, the role homeopathy can play, and parental rights; www.center4cby.com.
- Brennan, Patty. *Whole Family Recipes: For the Childbearing Year & Beyond;* whole foods cookbook with recipes your family will actually eat; www.center4cby.com.
- Castro, Miranda. *Homeopathy for Pregnancy, Birth, and Babies;* treatments for common ailments, including complementary support measures in addition to homeopathy.
- Chamberlain, David. *The Mind of Your Newborn Baby.*
- Cortlund, Lucke, and Miller Watelet. *Mother Rising: The Most Complete Guide to Blessingways.*
- England and Horowitz. *Birthing from Within;* use of birth art to process fears and emotions as preparation for birth.
- Fallon, Nancy. *Nourishing Traditions: The Cookbook that Challenges Politically Correct Nutrition and the Diet Dictocrats.*
- Gabriel, Cynthia. *Natural Hospital Birth: The Best of Both Worlds;* recommended.
- Gaskin, Ina May. *Ina's May Guide to Childbirth;* highly recommended.
- Goer and Romano. *Optimal Care in Childbirth: The Case for a Physiologic Approach.*
- Kitzinger, Sheila. *The Complete Book of Pregnancy and Childbirth, Revised Edition;* great overview includes psychological aspects; very down-to-earth author.
- La Leche League. *The Womanly Art of Breastfeeding, 8th Edition;* time-honored classic.
- Liedloff, Jean. *The Continuum Concept.*
- Lothian and DeVries. *The Official Lamaze Guide: Giving Birth with Confidence, 2nd Edition.*
- Maser, Shari. *Blessingways: A Guide to Mother-Centered Baby Showers.*
- Mendelsohn, Robert. *How to Raise a Healthy Child in Spite of Your Doctor;* for a consumer approach to pediatric care; highly recommended.
- Mohrbacher and Kendall-Tackett. *Breastfeeding Made Simple: Seven Natural Laws for Nursing Mothers.*
- Mongan, Marie. *HypnoBirthing: The Mongan Method* (comes with audio CD).
- Noble, Elizabeth. *Essential Exercises for the Childbearing Year;* includes a full chapter on the pelvic floor.
- Panuthos, Claudia. *Transformation through Birth;* great material on the emotional and psychological aspects of birth; good for processing fears and past trauma.
- Romm, Aviva Jill. *The Natural Pregnancy Book: Herbs, Nutrition and Other Holistic Choices;* website is a reliable source of information on safe use of herbs in pregnancy and while breastfeeding from an MD-herbalist; www.AvivaRomm.com.

- Romm, Aviva Jill. *Natural Healing After Birth: The Complete Guide to Postpartum Wellness.*
- Sears Library. *The Baby Book: Everything You Need to Know about Your Baby from Birth to Age Two, Revised Edition;* www.askdrsears.com.
- Sears, Robert. *The Vaccine Book: Making the Right Decision for Your Child;* essentially pro-vaccine doctor discusses safety concerns regarding each vaccine and how to minimize risks.
- Simkin, Penny. *The Birth Partner: A Complete Guide to Childbirth for Dads, Doulas, and All Other Labor Companions, 4th Edition.*
- Simkin, Penny, et al. *Pregnancy, Childbirth, and the Newborn: The Complete Guide, 5th Edition;* excellent overview by acclaimed childbirth author.
- Tully, Gail. *The Belly Mapping Workbook;* empowers mothers to determine their baby's position in the womb; website contains really useful information for turning babies who are not optimally positioned prior to the birth; www.SpinningBabies.com.
- Weed, Susan. *Wise Woman Herbal for the Childbearing Year;* good self-help manual with reliable information for resolving discomforts of pregnancy.

## DVDs

- Klaus, Kennell, and Klaus. *The Amazing Talents of the Newborn*; also available in book form, but the DVD is especially fun (and instructive!) to watch.
- Karp, Harvey. *The Happiest Baby on the Block;* demonstrates a sequence of steps to calm a crying infant; I prefer the DVD to the book; if pressed for time (the whole program is one hour long), skip to sections on "The Fourth Trimester" and "The Five S's."

## Best of the Web

Please email patty@center4cby.com for a free download (PDF) that includes recommended websites for childbearing couples. That way, I can provide you with easy access to all the links.